INTERMITTENT FASTING DIET FOR WOMEN OVER 50

Unlock The Key For A Healthy Weight Loss With The Most Complete Guide For Beginners And Diabetics Packed With Practical Tips | Weekly Meal Plan Included

Table of Contents

Introduction

Intermittent fasting (IF) is just a method for partitioning your meal plans into times of eating and fasting.

Intermittent fasting for women over 50 has been clinically demonstrated to upgrade the skeletal framework's overall well-being. It has been seen as a productive method for diminishing the indications of joint inflammation and back agony, which more seasoned women usually experience. A couple of studies have additionally demonstrated how changing meal plans as per IF can influence the generation of hormones that control muscle and bone wellbeing.

For women over 50, this method can also help expand confidence and better mind-sets alongside a reduction in negative manifestations like uneasiness, despair, and stress.

Eating during specific timeframes is associated with a diminished danger of diabetes. A few investigations show that intermittent fasting can be a productive method to hold glucose levels under tight restraints, get off insulin, and even dispose of or decrease the use of recommending medications.

When a woman begins fasting at fixed interims, her body begins sending a sign that actuates a hereditary fix instrument. This system battles maturing and different sicknesses by delivering human development hormone (HGH). Thus, HGH attempts to strengthen muscles, tendons, and ligaments, accelerate metabolic rate, recover tissues, and increment life span. This is ostensibly probably the best bit of leeway of intermittent fasting for women over 50.

Being perhaps the most sizzling theme in the weight loss world, intermittent fasting has substantiated itself as a fruitful solution for getting thinner, keeping up bulk, expanding life span, and in any event, upgrading discernment. Most importantly, it is considered broadly valuable for more established women who need to lose paunch fat.

Chapter 1: What is Intermittent Fasting and its Types

Intermittent fasting is an eating pattern where a person cycles between eating and fasting periods. Therefore, it is more of a way of eating than a diet.

Intermittent fasting is not as hard as you may think. If anything, it is the exact opposite. There is less planning involved, and many people who have practiced it say that they feel more energetic and generally good during the fast. It may be challenging when starting, but the body quickly adapts, and you get used to it.

Types of Intermittent Fasting

16/8 Method

This's just about the most popular fasting methods since it's so schedule-based, meaning there are no surprises. This will give you the freedom to control when you eat based on the everyday life of yours. The sixteen is the number of hours you're likely to be fasting, which may also be lowered to twelve or perhaps fourteen hours if that fits into your life better. Then your eating period is going to be between eight and ten hours every day. This might seem daunting, but it just means that you are skipping an entire meal. Many people choose to begin their fast around 7 or 8 p.m. and then do not eat until 11 or noon the next day, which means they fast for the recommended 16 hours. Of course, it isn't as bad as it sounds since they are sleeping during this time, so what it comes down to is eating dinner and then not eating again the next day around lunch, so you are just skipping breakfast.

You will be doing it every day, so finding the hours that work for you are important. If you work the third shift, then switching your eating period to fit into your schedule is important. If you find yourself running down and sluggish, tweak your fasting hours until you find a healthy balance. Granted, there will be some adjustment, because, chances are, your body is not accustomed to skipping entire meals. However, this should go away after a couple of weeks. If it doesn't then try starting your fasting period earlier in the day, allowing you to eat earlier or alter it, you need to feel healthy and happy.

Lean-Gains Method (14:10)

The lean-gains method has several different incarnations on the web, but its fame comes from the fact that it helps shed fat while building it into muscle almost immediately. Through the lean-gains method, you'll find yourself able to shift all that fat to be muscle through a rigorous practice of fasting, eating right, and exercising.

Through this method, you fast anywhere from 14 to 16 hours and spend the remaining 10 or 8 hours each day engaged in eating and exercise. As opposed to the crescendo, this method features daily fasting and eating, rather than alternated eating days versus not. Therefore, you don't have to be quite cautious about extending the physical effort to exercise on the days you are fasting because those days when you're fasting are every day!

For the lean-gaining method, start fasting only for 14 hours and work it up to 16 if you feel comfortable with it, but never forget to drink enough water and be careful about spending too much energy on exercise! Remember that you want to grow in health and potential through intermittent fasting. You'll certainly not want to lose any of that growth by forcing the process along.

20:4 Method

Stepping things up a notch from the 14:10 and 16:8 methods, the 20:4 method is a tough one to master, for it is rather unforgiving. People talk about this method of intermittent fasting as intense and highly restrictive. Still, they also say that the effects of living this method are almost unparalleled with all other tactics.

For the 20:4 method, you'll fast for 20 hours each day and squeeze all your meals, all your eating, and all your snacking into 4 hours. People who attempt 20:4 normally have two smaller meals or just one large meal and a few snacks during their 4-hour window to eat, and it is up to the individual which four hours of the day they devote to eating.

The trick for this method is to make sure you're not overeating or bingeing during those 4-hour windows to eat. It is all-too-easy to get hungry during the 20-hour fast and have that feeling then propel you into intense and unrealistic hunger or meal sizes after the fast period is over. Be careful if you try this method. If you're new to intermittent fasting, work your way up to this one gradually, and if you're working your way up already, only make the shift to 20:4 when you know you're ready. It would surely disappoint if all your progress with intermittent fasting got hijacked by one poorly thought-out goal with 20:4 method.

Meal Skipping

Meal skipping is an extremely flexible form of intermittent fasting that can provide all of the benefits of intermittent fasting but with a less strict schedule. If you are not someone who has a typical schedule or feels like a more strict variation of the intermittent fasting diet will serve you, meal skipping is a viable alternative.

Many people who choose to use meal skipping find it a great way to listen to their bodies and follow their basic instincts. If they are not hungry, they simply don't eat that meal.

Instead, they wait for the next one. Meal skipping can also help people who have time constraints and who may not always get in a certain meal of the day.

It is important to realize that you may not always be maintaining a 10–16-hour window of fasting with meal skipping. As a result, you may not get every benefit that comes from other fasting diets. However, this may be a great solution for people who want an intermittent fasting diet that feels more natural. It may also be a great idea for those looking to begin listening to their bodies more so that they can adjust to a more intense variation of the diet with greater ease. It can be a great transitional diet for you if you are not ready to jump into one of the other fasting diets just yet.

Warrior Diet Fasting

The most extreme form of intermittent fasting is known as the Warrior Diet. This intermittent fasting cycle follows a 20-hour fasting window with a short 4-hour eating window. During that eating window, individuals are supposed only to consume raw fruits and vegetables. They can also eat one large meal. Typically, the eating window occurs at nighttime so people can snack throughout the evening, have a large meal, and then resume fasting.

Because of the fasting length of the Warrior Diet, people should also consume a fairly hearty level of healthy fats. Doing so will give the body something to consume during the fast to produce energy with. A small number of carbohydrates can also be incorporated to support energy levels, too.

People who eat the Warrior Diet tend to believe that humans are natural nocturnal eaters and are not meant to eat throughout the day. The belief is that eating this way follows our natural circadian rhythms, allowing our body to work optimally.

The only people who should consider doing the Warrior Diet have already had success with other forms of intermittent fasting and who are used to it. Attempting to jump straight into the Warrior Diet can have serious repercussions for anyone who is not used to intermittent fasting. Even still, those used to it may find this particular style too extreme for them to maintain.

Eat-Stop-Eat (24 Hour) Method

This method of fasting is incredibly similar to the crescendo method. The only discernable difference is that there's no anticipation of increasing into a more intense fasting pattern with time. For the eat-stop-eat method, you decide which days you want to take off from eating, and then you run with it until you've lost that weight and then keep running with the lifestyle for good because you won't be able to imagine life without it.

The eat-stop-eat method involves one to two days a week being 100% oriented towards fasting, with the other five to six days concerning "business as normal." The one or two days spent fasting are then full 24-hour days spent without eating anything at all. These days, of course, water and coffee are still fine to drink, but no food items can be consumed whatsoever. Exercise is also frowned upon on those fasting days but see what your body can handle before deciding how that should all work out.

Some people might start thinking they're using the crescendo method but end up sticking with eat-stop-eat.

Alternate-Day Method

The alternate-day method is admittedly a little confusing, but the reason it could be so confusing could come, in part, from how much wiggle room it provides for the practitioner.

This method is great for people who don't have a consistent schedule or any sense of one, it is incredibly forgiving for those who don't quite have everything together for themselves yet.

When it comes down to it, alternate-day intermittent fasting is really up to you. You should try to fast every other day, but it doesn't have to be that precise. Similarly, with the crescendo method, as long as you fast two to three days a week, with a break day or two in between each fasting day, you're set! Then, you'll want to eat normally for three or four days out of each week, and when you encounter a fasting day, you don't even need to completely fast!

Alternate-day fasting is a solid place to start from, especially if you work a varying schedule or still have to get used to a consistent one. If you want to make things more intense from this starting point, the alternate-day method can easily become the eat-stop-eat method, the crescendo method, or the 5:2 method. Essentially, this method is a great place to begin.

12:12 Method

As another of the more natural ways of intermittent fasting, 12:12 approach is well-suited to beginning practitioners. Many people live out 12:12 method without any forethought simply because of their sleeping and eating schedule but turning 12:12 into a conscious practice can have just as many positive effects on your life as the more drastic 20:4 method claims.

According to a study conducted in the University of Alabama For this method, you fast for 12 hours and then enter a 12-hour eating window. It's not difficult to get three small meals and several snacks, or two big meals and a snack into your day with this method. With the 12:12 method, the standard meal schedule works well.

Ultimately, this method is a great one to start from, for a lot of variation can be built into this scheduling when you're ready to make things more interesting. Effortlessly and without much effort, 12:12 can become 14:10 or even 16:8, and in seemingly no time, you can find yourself trying alternate-day or crescendo methods, too. Start with what's normal for you, and this method might be exactly that!

Chapter 2: Why IF Is Good for Women Over 50

Boost Weight Loss

Most people discover intermittent fasting either because they want to lose weight or gain health benefits. But, sometimes losing weight can accomplish both of those simultaneously, as a high body fat percentage can increase high blood pressure, cholesterol, and early mortality. Whether you are hoping to gain these health benefits by losing weight or wish to lose weight to feel more comfortable in your skin, you will love how intermittent fasting can boost your weight loss.

Balance Important Hormones

Thankfully, studies have found intermittent fasting can help balance a person's cortisol and melioration levels. It does this in a variety of ways. For instance, it can help to reduce cortisol by balancing and regulating blood sugar levels. Balancing cortisol sets off a chain reaction that improves the balance of other hormones, including melatonin. One simple change can benefit many hormones and systems within your body.

Improve Heart Health

As we age, we all must take even more care of our heart health. After all, heart disease is the number one killer of both men and women. While doctors often educate men on the symptoms and warning signs of heart attacks, women are often forgotten, leading to an increased risk of death. This means women must be extra vigilant, taking care of their heart health and educating themselves on the warning signs of heart attacks.

One crucial way to increase heart health is to watch your cholesterol. There is not a single type of cholesterol, but several. The two main types include LDL, known as the "bad" cholesterol, and HDL, known as the "good" cholesterol. While LDL cholesterol will increase your heart attack and heart disease risk, HDL cholesterol will protect your heart and remove LDL cholesterol from your body.

Increase Mental Energy and Efficiency

We all need mental energy to get through the day. When our mind is sluggish, we cannot think, accomplish anything, and sometimes we may be unable even to stay awake. We have all had trouble focusing on work, completing a math problem, remembering what we have read, and so on. This is all due to a lack of mental energy and efficiency. You may think that intermittent fasting would further reduce your mental state, as hunger makes focusing difficult, but the opposite is exact.

Reduce the Potential Risk of Developing Cancer

Of course, nobody can promise that any lifestyle choice will prevent you from developing cancer. However, studies have found that intermittent fasting can potentially reduce your risk. Further studies are ongoing, but current research through animal studies have proven promising. For instance, it was found that rats with tumors survive longer when placed on fasting schedules than the control group.

Increase Longevity

Early studies on animals have found that an animal can experience an increased lifespan by including intermittent fasting. These studies found that even if animals had a higher body fat percentage than the control group, including intermittent fasting, they could increase their lifespan and longevity.

This makes sense, as intermittent fasting has many health benefits, and when all of these benefits are compounded together, it naturally results in a longer lifespan.

Lifestyle Ease

We all want to improve health and weight, but it is important also to have an easier lifestyle. When it is difficult to gain health and weight, many of us fail, as life is already busy and difficult enough without adding added worry and tasks. If a person cooks more, eats more frequently, and always worries about a diet, they are unlikely to stick to it, as it is merely unmaintainable.

It supports the secretion of the growth hormone

It's present in kids more than in grown-ups, but it still helps a lot. The growth hormone decreases fat and improves the development of bone and muscles. It does this by turning glycogen into glucose in the bloodstream. This enables fat burn without the reduction of muscles. When you sleep and exercise enough, the growth hormone is also boosted.

It enables you to avoid heart illnesses

Both blood glucose control and fat loss are done by IF to improve heart health. The likelihood of getting coronary artery heart illness can also be reduced.

Intermittent fasting is very versatile and can fit in any schedule

It is not as challenging as certain diets that unnecessarily trigger a huge disturbance in your life. There is no particular time to perform the IF. They can be blended as you think it is appropriate for your timetable. You are not boxed into any regiment that you cannot retain easily. Intermittent rapidity adapts to life's unpredictability. This can also be practiced everywhere globally as there is no special gear you need to do; it only restricts your feeding and is therefore much easier and more practical than many diets. It's completely all right, even if you have to halt fasting for a while. In a matter of minutes, you can begin fasting again.

It accepts all food

 Organic foods have more nutrients than processed foods. These organic products are unfortunately quite costly, so purchasing them will diminish your pockets every day. They can be almost 10 times more expensive than processed products. It is easier to afford processed products as they are cheap. No matter the effectiveness of a diet, it cannot help you if you can't afford it. Fasting is in the first position of cost-effectiveness since it is completely free. You don't have to purchase any meals, so it costs you no cash. There's no reason you purchase costly meals or supplements or any drug that makes it cheap for all.

Simple to practice

Intermediate fasting is easy to do and doesn't have any complicated scheduling, it is quite direct. This causes it to be simpler to pursue and more efficient than many diets.

Opens up your mind

It enables you to regulate your mental procedures as IF opens up your body. You are used to responding to your body's urges because you consume whenever you feel slightly hungry. You are released from the control of your body as a result of practicing IF.

Corrects insulin resistance

This is the simplest and easiest route to reduce insulin resistance and insulin levels. It has a highly effective impact. It works better than a rigid low-carb diet.

Improves your metabolism

Intermittent fasting enhances your metabolism by considerably reducing the number of calories you eat in one day. During the feeding time you have, it is almost possible to eat the suggested daily calorific requirements. This causes modifications in the body and fat burning. It also helps you burn fat, even if you eat the normal calories your system requires, as it will make you burn fat for power instead of carbs.

Chapter 3: IF and Hormones

Upon reaching the age of 30, the aging process starts, and the body's hormones fluctuate. The process is different for everyone depending on genetics and several environmental factors, as men and women have different phases in their lives that affect the levels of their hormones. The human growth hormone is produced by the pituitary gland and contributes to adolescents' growth and development. The deficiency of human growth hormone in an adult means higher body fat and reduced muscle mass and bone density. Once it is availed from the pituitary gland, the human growth hormone only lasts a short time in the blood. From there, it finds its way to the liver where it is metabolized and initiated into growth factors.

That would be the same, which is linked to high insulin levels that lead to several health issues. However, the brief instance of the growth factors from human growth hormone lasts only a few minutes. All of the hormones are secreted naturally and done so in brief bursts to prevent the initiation of some resistance, which happens when the body gets used to high levels of the hormone in the bloodstream without acting proportionately to their secretion. The first discoveries of human growth hormone came from experiments on cadavers done in the 50s though it was synthesized in a lab environment during the 80s. After that, it became very popular as a performance-enhancing supplement. The normal levels of the hormone in a person tend to reach a peak during puberty as expected, and they gradually decrease afterward. Growth hormone tends to be produced when a person is sleeping and is one of the counter-regulatory hormones produced naturally. Both cortisol and HGH increase the level of glucose in the bloodstream by breaking down the glycogen to counters the effects that are rendered by insulin. Insulin reduces the amount of blood glucose levels while HGH increases blood glucose.

These hormones are usually secreted in pulses before a person wakes up. This would be deemed normal and it is supposed to get the body ready for the day by pushing the glucose out of storage and into the bloodstream where it is then available for energy creation. When someone says that a person needs to eat their breakfast to have the right energy levels for the day, this is very incorrect. The body has already provided enough resources for this to happen so there is no need to do cereals or a heavy breakfast to get the fuel needed for the day. This is why hunger happens to be its lowest during the early morning even if someone has not eaten during the night unless the body has already been conditioned to consume food during this time, which happens with most people.

Fasting to Increase the Levels of the Growth Hormone

In 1982, Kerndt produced a study that was of a single patient and they went through a 40-day fast for religious needs. The glucose levels decreased, from a level of 96, it dropped to a level of 56. The insulin went much lower and stabilized. The concern was the HGH though. According to the study, it started at a level of 0.74 and peaked at 9.86. That would mean a 1,250% increase in the level of the growth hormone. Even a fast for five days gives a significant increase in the growth hormone.

This is all according to research done on the subject. The question then goes to the potential side effects of the increased growth hormone from fasting. There might be an increased level of blood sugar for someone but there is hardly a risk for the potential of debilitating lifestyle diseases such as cancer and diabetes.

Fasting is seen as one of the great stimulating factors for HGH secretion. During the time of fasting, there happens to be a spike during the morning period, but there is usually some secretion going on during the day. The HGH is crucial after all to maintain and develop muscle fiber and bone density. Though, some of the main issues that come with fasting include the decreased levels of muscle mass. Some say fasting a single day would even cause a loss of about ¼ of a pound of muscle. The opposite is said to happen according to verified research. In comparing the caloric reduction diets to fasting, the fasting was much better at preserving lean mass.

Say that somebody is living during the prehistoric Paleolithic era. During the summer when food is abundant, the community would engage in a lot of feasting and then store some of that as fat within the body. During the time of winter, there would be nothing to eat. The question is whether the body would metabolize the muscle but preserve the stored fat. In this case, the body would burn the stored fat instead of the precious muscle fiber. It is true though that some protein is catabolized for gluconeogenesis purposes, though the increase in HGH maintains lean mass during the time of fasting.

The increases in human growth hormone when a person is fasting assist in preserving the muscle tissue and glycogen stores while using the fat stores instead. This breakdown of the fat in a process known as lipolysis releases glycerol and other fatty acids, which would be metabolized to create energy. Madelon Buijs, a researcher at the Leiden University Medical Center in the Netherlands, claims the increases in HGH rise noticeably during the first 13 hours of beginning a fast, which would mean an increased breakdown of fats in the first half of the day of the fast.

Blood Levels of Human Growth Hormone

When fasting, loss of protein from the muscles increases by 50 percent in the cases of a lack of human growth hormone. Though, fasting and exercise during the fast may increase the levels of growth hormone. They are also subject to a lot of variation during the day because the pituitary gland releases the hormone in particular bursts. The random evaluation of the levels of human growth hormone as opposed to monitoring it overtime is not necessarily useful. Though, levels during the morning would be much higher than those recorded during the day.

Implications for the Athletes

This has significant ramifications for the athletes as it is known as training during the fasting phase. The increase of adrenaline from fasting will increase motivation so that the person will train harder. Similarly, the increased HGH levels as stimulated by the intermittent fasting will result in a toning effect and an increase in muscle mass that will help make recovery from the workout sessions that much easier. That would be a significant advantage for the athletes, especially in the endurance department. There is also a lot of new attention given to this approach to muscle treatment and exercise. It is not luck that many of the early proponents in training during the fasting state are bodybuilders. This is because it is a sport that requires a lot of high-intensity training and very low levels of body fat.

Even a book was written by bodybuilder Brad Pilon known as 'Eat, Stop, Eat'—which popularized the lean gains approach to fasting. For those individuals who believed fasting would increase fatigue levels and make you tired or it would not be possible to exercise during fasting, that is a wrong mentality. Fasting in itself does not cause you to burn muscle fiber significantly. There is no typical approach, meaning you have to shrivel up into a skeleton to get effective results from the fasted state. The difference with those scenarios is the individuals illustrated did not receive any form of nourishment during their fasts. They could even go weeks without sufficient water and food between days. At that level, you would be punishing your body rather than taming it and the situations are due to lack rather than an active choice because no one can hold out that long.

As such, fasting when done right has good potential in creating anti-aging properties brought about by human growth hormone without the potential problems created by excess HGH such as increased blood pressure and prostate cancer. For those interested in competing at an elite or athletic level, then the benefits would be much better for them.

Additional Information

The testing that comes with HGH is not particularly routine. At times, it is done to help diagnose the pituitary issues that can sometimes lead to conditions like gigantism or stunted growth. Even though HGH therapy is approved when it comes to treating those children that have stunted growth, it has also attracted a lot of attention because of the effects that it has been deemed to have on muscle and fat tissues. Synthetic HGH is available for purchase though not a lot is known about the long-term safety it has on the subject.

Chapter 4: Setting Goals

Set Goals

A healthy weight loss goal is to lose between one and two pounds every week. If you start losing more, there's a chance that you are losing muscle mass. There's credible research to confirm that it's possible to lose lean muscle mass with Intermittent Fasting if you don't eat enough protein. You can be healthy when it comes to weight but still have high amounts of abdominal fat, which can cause many health risks. The goals with Intermittent Fasting depend on your health and weight goals. You can determine your diet goals by answering a couple of simple questions:

Which improvements are you seeking? Do you want to:

- Reduce the symptoms of illness,
- Feel better,
- Become more energized,
- Lose weight, or
- All of the above?
- Are you interested in practicing the diet long-term, or only until you meet your goals?
- How will you track the intake of macronutrients?
- What are your diet preferences?

Calculate Body Mass Index

Body Mass Index or BMI is an indicator of whether your current weight is healthy compared to your height. You can calculate your BMI by dividing your weight in kilograms by your squared height (m). If your results are between 18.5 and 24.9, you are healthy. Anything below 18.5 isn't healthy. The ideal measure is 21 for women and 23 for men. However, this calculation doesn't account for body fat, waist circumference, eating habits, and lifestyle. All of this goes into how healthy you are.

Your BMI can be higher if you are masculine, which doesn't mean that you should lose weight if you are healthy. You can think of yourself as obese if your BMI is over 30. However, this isn't exclusive to the number because it's possible to have a healthy weight with an unhealthy body fat. These are rough calculations that can cause you to think of Athletic and someone who is thinner but has more body fat as obese. However, calculating your BMI can help you determine your weight loss goals in collaboration with your doctor and a dietitian.

Calculate the Body Fat Percentage

Looking into your body-fat percentage will help you to understand what you should do to lose weight, for example:

- Which method of Intermittent Fasting is the most appropriate?

- Whether or not you want to incorporate the Keto diet in Intermittent Fasting?

- How much do you need to exercise, and what kind of exercises are necessary?

If you like exercising, Intermittent Fasting will help you lose body fat, but preserve or gain muscle mass. As a result, you may not notice scaling down. However, even if you don't lose weight, but gain muscle mass, you will still look slimmer.

To track how your body fat changes, you can use the body composition scales. These scales help you track how your muscle mass, your hydration, and your body fat change throughout your diet.

Calculate Waist-to-Hip Ratio

The waist-hip ratio or WHR is a more credible measurement because it accounts for your natural body shape. For women, an ideal measure is 0.8, while 0.9 is ideal for men. If your measurements are higher, you should work on your shape.

For calculating the WHR, you can use a tape measure and measure the circumference of the widest part of your hips and your natural waist, which is slightly above your belly button. After that, divide your waist measurement by your hip measurement.

Plan Your Portions

Calculate Basal Metabolic Rate

While measuring meals isn't required with Intermittent Fasting, it is desirable to maintain optimal health levels. To start, you should calculate your basal metabolic rate to find out how many calories you need to maintain your weight, and how many you need to lose it.

Calculate the Right Portion Sizes

When calculating portion sizes, keep in mind that 1 gram of nutrients translates to a different number of calories:

- Fat-9 calories,

- Protein- 4 calories, and

- Carbohydrate-4 calories.

Calculate the Daily Calorie Intake

In general, Intermittent Fasting doesn't require calorie restriction for weight loss. Still, weight loss and other health benefits of fasting will be greater if you have a controlled daily calorie intake.

Chapter 5: Rules to Follow to Lose Weight

It is very important to reiterate that proper transition into an intermittent fasting lifestyle is very important.

It is a Lifestyle Change

A very important thing that people easily and most often overlook is that intermittent fasting is just not staying hungry for a few hours a day. It is a complete lifestyle change. As you are reading this book, you might find it very easy. It can't be too difficult to stay hungry for 12-16 hours. Believe me; it isn't. However, when you need to respect that limitation for months and years, it can look difficult. Most people don't go that far. They start finding it difficult within a week or a month at the most.

Eliminating snacks from your routine will be the hardest decision you'll make. Not having anything voluntarily and not being able to have anything are two very different things.

Most people fail in their weight loss journey because first, they believe that things are very easy and then come under the impression that they are very difficult. The truth lies somewhere in-between.

1. You must start with the elimination of snacks.

2. Follow this routine for so long that you don't feel the need to have snacks

3. Then, begin placing three nutrient-dense meals within an eating window of 12 hours

4. Follow this routine until you're are well adjusted to it.

5. Increase your fasting hours to 14.

6. Follow this routine for at least a quarter

7. Begin shifting your breakfast as closer to lunch as possible without putting too much strain on your body

8. At this stage, you must not set a goal for fasting hours. Just don't eat as long as you don't feel really hungry

9. You must also keep in mind not to starve yourself when feeling hungry

10. Only stick to a longer fast if you are comfortable with it and never rush with any step on the way

It Only Looks Easy

This is very important learning you must keep with yourself. Intermittent fasting only looks easy, but it is a lifestyle that needs to be practiced. Even with intermittent fasting, you will experience frustrating moments when you wouldn't want to move ahead. You must never take it for granted.

Following a routine with discipline is difficult, and training yourself to follow it with precision is always a challenge. If you want to succeed in your goals, you must plan.

How to Plan

Step One – Create a Monthly Calendar

On a calendar, highlight the days you wish to fast, depending on the type of fast you have committed yourself to. Record a start and end time on your fasting days, so you know how you plan to begin and finish in the days leading up to your fast day.

Tick off your days; this will keep you motivated and on track!

Step Two – Record Your Findings

Create a journal for your fasting journey. One or two days before the time, undertake to do your measurements. Weigh yourself first thing in the morning, after you have gone to the restroom, and before breakfast. Also, do not weigh yourself wearing heavy items as they may affect the outcome of the scale.

Measure your height as this figure is related to your BMI (body mass index) result.

Record the measurements around your hips and stomach area, if you wish, you can also measure your upper thighs and arms.

Take a photo of yourself and place it into the journal too; this is not to discourage you but to keep you focused on why you began this journey.

Jot down all of these findings and update them weekly in the journal.

A journal is also the perfect way to express how you are feeling and, of course, what you are most thankful for. A journal is an important way to track not just the physical aspects of the diet but also its mental aspects. Never undertake to doubt yourself; your journal should be a safe space for you to congratulate and to motivate yourself. Leave all the negative thoughts at the door!

Step Three – Plan Your Meals

The easiest way to stick to any eating program is to plan your meals; 500 calorie meals tend to be simple and easy to create but there are also many other more complex recipes for those who wish to spice things up. Who knows, perhaps you stumble across a meal you wish to eat outside of your fasting days.

It is advised that you prepare your meals the day before your fast days; doing this helps you stay committed to the fast and limits food wastage.

Initially, and in the first few weeks, it is suggested that you keep your meal preparation and recipes simple, so as not to overcomplicate the whole process. This also allows you to get used to counting your calories and knowing which foods work to keep you fuller versus those that left you feeling hungrier earlier than later.

Be sure to include your meal plan in your journal and on your calendar.

Step Four – Reward Yourself

On the days where you may return to normal eating, it is important to reward yourself. A small reward goes a long way in reminding yourself and your brain that what you are doing has merit and that it should be noticed.

A reward should cater to one of our primal needs; these needs include:

- Self-actualization

- Safety needs

- Social needs

- Esteem needs

Physiological needs such as food, water, air, clothing, and shelter.

Have a block of chocolate or buy yourself a new item of clothing to do anything that makes your heart happy!

Step Five – Curb Hunger Pains

Initially, you will feel more discomfort when hungry, but these feelings will pass. If you do find yourself craving something, sip on black tea or coffee to help you through your day. Coffee is known to alleviate the feelings of being hungry; if you must add sweetener, do so at your discretion. Know that some sweeteners can cause the opposite effect and make you feel hungry.

Step Six – Stay busy

Keeping busy means that the mind does not have time to dwell on your current state of affairs, especially if you find yourself reaching for a snack bar or cookie.

It is also wise to be implementing some sort of physical activity, even on your fasting days. A 20-minute walk before ending your fasting period will do wonders to help you reach the final stages of the fasting period. It can also uplift your mood when you are feeling frustrated or tense.

Step Seven – Practice Mindful Eating

As mentioned, we are inclined to eat for all sorts of reasons; happy, sad, it does not matter. The problem is that these feelings related to food become habitual, so we aren't really hungry, but we seek to tuck into something delicious because we feel good or even off.

The art of eating mindfully is not to allow these habits to master your life. The concept is simple: teach yourself to look at something, for instance, a piece of cake and think, "Do I need it or do I want it for other reasons?" You could decide to have a bite or two and leave the rest, but you may be less inclined to eat the whole slice (or whole cake) if you think mindfully about it.

The art of mindful eating is to revel in the food placed before you. Pay attention to colors, textures, and tastes. Savor each bite, even when eating an apple.

Your brain gradually begins to rewire itself when it comes to food and when it needs or wants something.

Practice mindful eating by:

- Pay attention to where your food comes from.

- Listen to what your body is telling you; stop eating when you are full.

- Only eat when your body signals you to do so; when your stomach growls or if you feel faint or if your energy levels are low.

- Pay attention to what is both healthy and unhealthy for us.

- Consider the environmental impact our food choices make.

- Every time you take a bite of your meal, set your cutlery down.

Step Eight – Practice Portion Control

Controlling portion sizes can be difficult for most; society has also regulated us to what we think is the size of an average portion. We have access to supersizing meals too, which does not help those struggling in the weight department. In 1961, Americans consumed 2,880 calories per day; by 2017, they consumed 3,600 calories, which is a 34% increase and an unhealthy one at that.

To help you navigate how to portion your food better, consider trying the following: when dishing up your food, try the following trick. Half of your plate should consist of healthy fruits and/or vegetables, one quarter should be made up of your starches such as potatoes, rice, or pasta, and the remaining quarter should be made up of lean meats or seafood.

Alternatively, try the following:

- Dish up onto a smaller plate or into a smaller bowl.

- Say no to upsizing a meal if offered.

- Buy the smaller version of the product if available or divide the servings equally into packets.

- Eat half a meal at the restaurant and take the remaining half to enjoy the following day instead.

- Go to bed early; it will stop any after-dinner eating.

Step Nine – Get Tech Savvy

Modern-day society has plenty to offer us in terms of the apps we can use to help determine the steps we take, the calories we burn, the calories found in our foods, research, information, and motivation for lifestyle changes, especially diets and exercise. The list is endless. There are many apps on the market currently that can help you track your progress in fasting.

The best intermittent fasting apps currently (at the time of writing), and in no particular order are:

- Zero

- Fast Habit

- Body Fast

- Fasting

- Vora

- Ate Food Diary

Life Fasting Tracker

Make use of your mobile device to set reminders for yourself when to eat, what to eat, and when your fast days are. It works especially well when using it to set reminders when you should drink water, particularly for those who find it hard to keep their fluids up.

Making the Change

Understand that intermittent fasting is not a diet; it is a lifestyle, an eating plan that you are in control of, and one that is easy to perfect. Before you know it, fasting will become second nature.

When to Start?

Begin today, not tomorrow or after a particular event or gathering. Once you have picked the fast that best suits you, begin with it immediately. Never hold off until a specific day; once you begin, you will gain momentum and it will become something that is part of your day, like many other things that fill up your day. No sweat there!

Measure Your Eating

Three days before you fast, it would be wise to begin to lessen the amount of food you are eating or dishing up less. This helps your body begin to get used to the idea that it doesn't need a whole bowl of food to get what it needs or feel full.

Keep up Your Exercise Plan

If you have a pre-existing exercise regime, do not alter it anyway. Simply carry on the way you were before fasting. If you are new to exercising, begin with short walks now and again, extending the time you walk. For example, take a five-minute walk, and the next day, change the time to 10 minutes of walking.

Stop, Start, Stop

Fast for hours, and then eat all your calories during a certain number of hours. Consider this as a training period.

Do Your Research

Read up as much as you can about intermittent fasting this way, it will put to rest any uncertainties you might have and introduce you to new ways of getting through a fasting day. Check out recipes that won't make you feel like a rabbit having to chew on carrots all day if you are stuck with ideas of what to eat.

Have Fun

Lastly, have fun, and see what your body can do, even over 50. It is important to know that just because you are a certain age doesn't mean you are incapable of pursuing a new lifestyle change. Reward yourself when it is due, track your progress, adjust where the need is, and get your beauty sleep. This is another secret to achieving overall wellness and happiness.

Know Your BMI

Your BMI is based on your weight and height; thus, you can easily determine your body mass index, or BMI as it is more commonly known.

In total, there are four categories that an individual can fall into based on this figure. That is underweight, healthy, overweight, and obese. The concept is simple: our BMI gives us quantifiable amounts when comparing our height with our fat, muscles, bones, and organs.

How to Calculate Your BMI

To calculate your BMI, equate your weight (lbs.) x 703 divided by your height (in).

Once you have calculated your BMI, you can compare it to the body mass index chart to determine which category you are classed into.

Class	Your BMI Score
Underweight	less than 18.5 points
Normal weight	18.5 – 24.9 points
Overweight	25 – 29.9 points
Class 1 — Obesity	30 – 34.9 points
Class 2 — Obesity	35 – 39.9 points

Class 3 — Extreme obesity	40 + points

Chapter 6: Myths to Disprove About Intermittent Fasting

Issues that are not popular can be misunderstood with a lot of misconceptions and myths surrounding them. Intermittent fasting is one such issue. Many people with half-baked information suddenly become experts on the topic and are always willing to advise anyone willing to listen. It doesn't matter how long a false premise is considered correct, once the evidence is present, the error is exposed, and wise people will know to stick with the facts.

Myth 1: Intermittent Fasting is Unsafe for Older Adults

Anyone can engage in intermittent fasting as long as they do not have any medical conditions and are not pregnant or lactating. Of course, our bodies do not all have the same tolerance levels even in people that look exactly alike. If one or more persons respond negatively to intermittent fasting because they are advanced in age and are women, it does not mean that another will react the same way.

There is no doubt that intermittent fasting is not meant for everyone. Fasting is not safe for children because they need all the food they can get for continual development. Fasting in itself is not an issue for older people – any adult can fast.

Myth 2: You Gain Weight as You Age

A myth is a combination of facts and falsehood. This is a typical example of that. It is saying that growing older means your metabolism will slow down and your body will not burn or use up calories as fast as when you were younger. However, weight gain in older adults is not a given. The key to keeping your body performing optimally is to develop and maintain healthy habits such as fasting intermittently, drinking enough water, reducing stress levels, and getting adequate exercise.

Myth 3: Your Metabolism Slows Down During Fasting

This myth represents one of those big misunderstandings I mentioned earlier. The difference between calorie restriction and deliberately choosing when to take in calories is huge. Intermittent fasting does not necessarily limit calorie intake neither does it make you starve. It is when a person starves or under-eats that changes occur in their metabolic rate. But there is no change whatsoever in your metabolism when you delay eating for a few hours by fasting intermittently.

Myth 4: You Will Get Fat if You Skip Breakfast

"Breakfast is the most important meal of the day!" This is one of the more popular urban myths about intermittent fasting. It is in the same category with the myths, "Santa doesn't give you presents if your naughty," and "carrots give you night vision." Some people will readily point to a relative or friend who is fat because they don't eat breakfast. But the question is: are they fat because they don't eat breakfast? Or do they skip breakfast because they are fat and want to reduce their calorie intake?

The best way to collect unbiased data when conducting scientific studies is through randomized controlled trials (RTC). After a careful study of 13 different RTCs on the relationship weight gain and eating or skipping breakfast, researchers from Melbourne, Australia found that both overweight and normal-weight participants who ate breakfast gained more weight than participants who skipped breakfast. The researchers also found that there's a higher rate of calorie consumption later in the day in participants who ate breakfast.

This puts a hole in the popular notion that skipping breakfast will make people overeat later in the day (Harvard Medical School, 2019).

The truth is, there is nothing spectacular about eating breakfast as far as weight management is concerned. There is limited scientific evidence disproving or supporting the idea that breakfast influences weight. Instead, studies only show that there is no difference in weight loss or gain when one eats or skips breakfast.

Myth 5: Exercise Is Harmful to Older Adults Especially While Fasting

No. It is not harmful to exercise while fasting. And no, exercise is not harmful to older adults, whether they are fasting or not. On the contrary, exercising during your fasting window helps to burn stored fats in the body. When you perform physical activities after eating, your body tries to burn off new calories that are ingested from your meal. But when you exercise on an empty or nearly empty stomach, your body burns fats that are stored already and keeps you fit.

What is harmful to older adults is not engaging in exercises at all. A lack of exercise or adequate physical activity in older adults is linked to diabetes, heart disease, and obesity among other health conditions.

Researchers from Harvard Medical School demonstrated in a landmark study that frail and older women could regain functional loss through resistance exercise (Harvard Medical School, 2007). For ten weeks, participants from a nursing home (100 women aged between 72 and 98) performed resistance exercises three times a week. At the end of 10 weeks, the participants could walk faster, further, climb more stairs, and lift a great deal of weight than their inactive counterparts. Also, a 10-year study of healthy aging by researchers with the MacArthur Study of Aging in America found that older adults (people between 70 and 80

44

years) can get physically fit whether or not they have been exercising at their younger age. The bottom line is, as long as you can move the muscles in your body, do it because it is safe and will only help you live a better and longer life.

Myth 6: Eating Frequently Reduces Hunger

There is mixed scientific evidence in this regard. Some studies show that eating frequently reduces hunger in some people. On the other hand, other studies show the exact opposite. Interestingly, at least one study shows no difference in the frequency of eating and how it influences hunger (US National Library of Medicine, 2013). Eating can help some people get over cravings and excessive hunger, but there is no shred of evidence to prove that it applies to everyone.

Myth 7: You Can't Teach an Old Dog New Tricks

The brain never stops learning neither does it stop developing at any age. New neural pathways are created when a person learns something new at any age. And with continued repetition, the neural pathways become stronger until the behavior is habitual. Older people are often more persistent and have a higher motivation than younger people when it comes to learning new things. Learning should be a lifelong pursuit and not an activity reserved for young people.

Don't allow anyone to convince you into believing that it is too late to learn new eating habits because you are in your golden years or are approaching it. It doesn't matter if you've never tried fasting you can still train your brain to make fasting a habit even in old age. Start small, make it a natural occurrence in everyday life, repeating until you get used to it, and your positive results aka glowing skin, improved energy will motivate you to make it into a lifestyle.

Myth 8: You Must Lose Weight during Intermittent Fasting

This myth is rooted in the hype that intermittent fasting has received in recent years. Unless done correctly, intermittent fasting may not yield weight loss benefits. For you to experience any significant loss in weight, you must ensure that you eat healthily during your eating window. Equally, it is important to stick to the fasting schedule. If you keep cheating and adjusting your fasting window to favor more eating time or you overeat during the eating window to compensate for lost meals, your chances of losing weight will be greatly diminished.

Myth 9: Your Body Will Go Into "Starvation Mode" If You Practice Intermittent Fasting

This myth is based on the misconception of what the starvation mode is and what triggers it. First of all, starvation is when your body senses that there is a significant drop in energy supply and reduces your metabolic rate. In simple terms, it is a reduction in the rate at which your body burns fat as a lack of food. This is an automatic response to conserve energy. It makes sense to reduce energy consumption if there is little to no supply of further energy coming from meals. In other words, if you stay away from food for too long, your body activates the starvation mode and significantly stops any further loss of body fat.

Having said that, intermittent fasting does not trigger the starvation mode. Instead, intermittent fasting helps to increase your metabolic activities. Meaning, your body can burn more fat when you fast for short periods. Starvation mode is only triggered when you engage in prolonged fasting over 48 hours, a practice I do not recommend for older adults.

Myth 10: An Aging Skin is Better Taken Care of with Anti-Aging Cream

This is not necessarily true. Brown spots, sagging skin, and wrinkles can indeed be reversed using expensive creams and topical treatments especially if a dermatologist prescribes them. These topical products exfoliate the top layer of your skin and make them appear smoother. However, that result (clear, smooth skin) is only a temporary effect.

A better way to look younger without any side effects is by activating autophagy. Engaging in mild stress-inducing activities such as intermittent fasting and exercising are the way. One key element to maintaining healthy skin is quenching your skin's thirst. Not drinking enough water can damage skin causing it to become dry, blemished, and lead to wrinkles. Drinking adequate amounts of water every day is the best approach to successfully "take the years off."

Myth 11: Fasting Deprives Your Brain of Adequate Dietary Glucose

Some people believe that your brain will underperform if you don't eat foods rich in carbohydrates. This myth is rooted in the notion that your brain uses only glucose as its fuel. But your brain doesn't use only dietary glucose for fuel. Some very low-carb diets can cause your body to produce ketone bodies from high-fat foods. Your brain can function well on ketone bodies. Continuous, intermittent fasting coupled with exercise can trigger the production of ketone bodies. Additionally, your body can also use a process known as gluconeogenesis to produce the sugar needed by your brain. This means that your body can effectively produce it on its own without you feeding it with just carbs.

Intermittent fasting does not interfere with brain function or its fuel or energy needs. However, because intermittent fasting is not suitable for everyone, if you feel shaky, dizzy, or extremely fatigued during fasting, consider talking with your doctor or reducing your fasting window.

Myth 12: Intermittent Fasting Will Make Older Adults Lose Their Muscle

First of all, it is stereotypical and largely incorrect to think of older people as frail. Frailty is not limited to just older adults and is a generalization of old age. Younger people can become frail if they suffer from a disabling chronic disease or have a poor diet. Scientists studied data from almost half a million people and found that middle-aged adults as young as 37 show signs of frailty (Mail Online, 2018).

Chapter 7: Intermittent Fasting and Working Out

If food is your source of fuel, should you be exercising without it?

There are some people who keep their workout routine quite basic, taking the idea of being active as taking a walk or cleaning their house. Then there are people who follow their gym workout routines planned out five to six days a week and never skip a workout. They get their cardio in daily and combine it with weights. Some even tend to think of themselves as full-on bodybuilders.

When you reach the point that all you want to do is be the fittest you can be and thrive off it, it is a wonderful thing. Suddenly, losing weight or maintaining your goal weight and physique isn't such a difficult thing to do, and you hardly ever feel like skipping a workout. Anyone with that type of mentality will find that losing weight is extremely easy and not at all a difficult task that waits for you either before or after work in the evening. It's, in fact, something to look forward to.

However, for the average individual, working out may not be so fun and easy to do. It may seem like something you dread thinking about from the early hours of the morning to the evening when you finally reach your hour of working out.

Now, for those who don't take their workouts too seriously, not eating before a workout, like in the morning once you wake up, will seem relatively easy. That is, if you're going to walk your dog or consider vacuuming your carpet as a workout. On the other hand, if you feel like you need your fuel for a workout, should you be planning your meals around it to suit your needs or try something different?

Exercising on an Empty Stomach

Since your body makes use of stored carbohydrates, otherwise known as glycogen, when working out to provide you with energy, you should know that there's no need to eat before working out. In fact, at some point, you may have heard that fasted workouts are much better for fat loss than working out after eating. Working out during a fasting period can help you burn up to 20% more fat than if you ate breakfast before a morning workout.

That's because, after fasting for eight to 12 hours, your body taps into its fat stores. So, when you're working out during your fasting period, you are burning fat instead of calories because your calories have already been depleted. This promotes a leaner body and provides you with all the energy you need to get through your workout.

If you feel like you're really struggling to work out on an empty stomach, consider cutting your fasting period, perhaps from 16 hours to 10 or 12 hours. You can also take BCAA's to provide you with a proper boost of energy for your workout. Finally, you can try drinking a cup of coffee 15 to 30 minutes before working out.

Anyone that feels they just can't work out on an empty stomach or feel weak when doing so should opt for a workout in the afternoon or before their last meal of the day.

Is There a Safe Way to Exercise While Intermittent Fasting?

If you're interested in working out while integrating intermittent fasting into your daily schedule, there are a few things to consider first.

Research has proven that exercising after eating before the digestion of food takes place is necessary for anyone suffering from metabolic syndrome or type 2 diabetes. In that same breath, research also suggests that exercising when fasting every day can affect the biochemistry of your muscles, along with your metabolism (Weatherspoon, 2018).

Since your glycogen stores are likely to be depleted after fasting, you are, once again, more able to burn fat as fuel instead of calories. While it is believed that we can burn more fat on an empty stomach, there is more to learn before you dive into your fasted workouts.

Intermittent fasting combined with exercising for an extended period isn't considered a good thing, according to Priya Khorana, PhD, the Columbian University nutrition educator. Studies also suggest that there is a big chance of your metabolism slowing down as a result of long-term fasting. However, it can help you burn more fat for a certain period at a time (Weatherspoon, 2018).

During fasting, you can burn more fat, but unless it is suited for you, you may not perform as well as you normally would during your workouts. During your fasting period, unless your diet accommodates your workout routine, you could lose muscle mass. You could potentially also be able to maintain your current muscle mass, yet not be able to build more muscle.

To ensure you're working out safely while fasting, you should keep a schedule of your day. With intermittent fasting, it's very important to make your workout as effective as possible during fasting. Consider when it is the right time to exercise. This, of course, will depend on the type of fasting method you're following. If you only have an 8-hour window to fuel up on food, you may want to work out before you break your fast. Anyone focused on performance and recovery should work out on an empty stomach on the 16:8 fasting method to achieve lean muscle mass and burn fat.

When working out, it doesn't matter what type of diet you're following, you must choose the diet that suits the macronutrients you take before you work out. Consider only doing strength workouts on the day after you consume a lot of carbs. With cardio or short bursts of high-intensive training, like HIIT, however, you can do this on a low-carb day.

The best way to look after your body during intermittent fasting, to build lean muscle and avoid injuries, is to eat a healthy, balanced, and fueling meal after your workout. After an intense strength training workout, it is necessary to fuel up on up to 20 grams of protein and an adequate amount of carbs in a 30-minute window after your workout.

Other than that, be sure to stay hydrated and drink plenty of water during the day, eat a high-protein meal directly after your workout, push your electrolytes, and above all else, listen to your body.

Chapter 8: Simple to Follow Exercises

Yet many may wonder if it's safe to exercise during an intermittent fast. With the body depleted of nutrients during a fast after all, would it be wise to put it through any more strain than it's already under? According to the data, exercise while undergoing a fast has a direct effect on metabolism and the body's level of insulin. Both are activated with one going up and the other going down as the body recalibrates and begins to burn fat rather than carbs. Engaging in the right kind of workout will help to speed up this process even more. Having that said, here are some exercises to give your intermittent fast a major boost.

Running/Treadmill

There is really nothing better to get the body's metabolic cylinders running than a good run. As soon as your feet hit the pavement (or the treadmill), your heart rate increases, and the blood starts to much more vigorously pump through your body. With your bodily processes instantly speeding up like this, it's really no wonder that your metabolism might speed up as well. And this is precisely the case when you engage in this type of exercise during a fast. But having that said, just keep in mind that you have to be careful not to overdo it. And in order to ensure that you have the best experience, it is recommended that you only run during the first few hours of your fast. That way your body still has plenty of additional resources left over from the last meal you had before your fast began. If for example, you began your fast at 10 PM on a Thursday night, you should be good to run around the block at 7 AM Friday morning without any trouble. It is not advisable however to overexert yourself at the very end of your fast. Although most could probably handle it, just to be on the safe side, you should keep your running hours locked into the first few hours of your fast. Every step you take causes hormones to alert your metabolic engines that you are up and quite literally running.

Weightlifting

If you are a weightlifter, or interested in becoming one—I have some good news for you. Lifting weights does not interfere with your fast! In fact, lifting weights during a fast can prove quite beneficial. As mentioned previously in this book, the very style of intermittent fasting is designed to prevent muscle loss during fasting periods, but having that said, a little weightlifting will help to shield your body from muscle loss even more. Because the truth is, we all lose muscle as we age and if we don't work at maintaining it through muscle lifting, we just might find that our muscle mass declining significantly through the years. Even more beneficial for those wishing to lose weight, lifting weights during an intermittent fast also quickens the pace of fat burn even more. Just think about it, during a fast your body has already switched to burning fat for its fuel, so when you grunt, struggle, and strain to lift those weights, guess what your body's tapping into for energy? All that fat you want to get rid of! Do I dare say—this is a win-win situation? It most certainly is!

Pushups

One of the most traditional exercises you could ever even consider would be that of the classic pushup. Pushups have been around forever and there is a reason for that—they are highly effective. By making use of gravity and your own body weight, the push-up gets the heart going while the muscles do overtime to push the body up off the floor by virtue of arm strength alone. These exercises if done moderately—say no more than 20 to 30 pushups during a fast—can be highly effective in boosting your metabolism to the max, allowing an even more rapid depletion of the body's fat stores. This is some good news that you could most certainly use!

Squats

This is another great exercise that seems absolutely made for intermittent fasting. Squats focus on your glutes, quads and other muscles like there is no tomorrow! This exercise keeps you going and keeps you strong! As you might imagine, squats consist of the participant bending their knees and squatting down toward the ground as if they are sitting on a chair. This bending motion gets the blood flowing to the thighs and begins rapidly burning fat deposits. If you need to target fat in the legs in particular, you might want to give this exercise a try.

Dips

Why yes—we would be remiss if we did not mention dips! And no, I'm not talking about the stuff you dip your chips in at the football game, I'm talking about high intensity, fat busing exercise that will burn fat, boost your metabolism and make sure your upper body stays nice and strong. These exercises are just about perfect for intermittent fasting as they get the blood flowing without making you too tired in the process.

Planks

Planks are a fairly common yet highly efficient exercise that can be done at home, at the gym, or just about any place you may be at the time. This exercise is also quite nuanced and flexible when it comes to adjusting the intensity and the area of focus. Planks tend to build up quite a bit of endurance too, which is most certainly good for someone who is undergoing a fast. It is best to engage in this exercise during the first few hours of your fast, but they can be done periodically throughout the rest of the fasting day as well.

Reverse Lunge

This exercise may look easy at first glance but don't be fooled. Reverse lunges are a high intensity workout that gets your metabolism going. And when done during a fast, it really kicks things into high gear. They are also good for getting your legs in tip top shape which is beneficial for just about every other aerobic exercise you could do.

Burpee

No, a burpee isn't what happens when you eat too many hot peppers. A bad joke maybe, but in all seriousness, there are many out there who are confused with what a burpee is and what it is not. The Burpee is a classic hybrid styled exercise that makes full use of cardio as well as resistance exercises, in order to maximize your metabolism. These exercises are pretty intensive, so if you are engaged in a less than 500 calorie fast day, you might want actually to have a low-calorie snack or other healthy option. Good choices for nutrition before this workout would be perhaps just a 1 hard-boiled egg, a salad, or maybe even a bowl of chicken broth. Either way, these workouts are sure to get your body running on all cylinders during your intermittent fast.

Chapter 9: Intermittent Fasting & Keto Diet – The Perfect Duo

The ketogenic diet offers many of the same benefits associated with intermittent fasting, and when done together, most people will experience significant health improvements, including not just weight loss. The ketogenic diet and intermittent fasting allow the body to move from a state where sugar is burned to a state where fat is burned (important flexibility, which in turn promotes optimal cell function and body systems). And although there is evidence that the two strategies work independently, I understand that the combination of the two strategies provides the best results overall.

There are at least two important reasons to favor the pulse approach. Insulin deactivates liver gluconeogenesis, that is, the production of glucose by the liver. When insulin is chronically suppressed for long periods, the liver begins to compensate for its lack by producing more glucose. As a result, your blood sugar starts rising even if you don't eat carbohydrates.

More importantly, in general many metabolic benefits associated with nutritional ketosis actually occur during the re-feeding phase. In the fasting phase, the removal of damaged cells and their contents occurs, but the real rejuvenation process takes place during refeeding. In other words, the cells and tissues are rebuilt, and their healthy state is restored when the intake of net carbohydrates increases. (Rejuvenation during re-feeding is also one of the reasons why intermittent fasting has so many benefits, because you cycle hunger and abundance.)

How to Apply Cyclic Ketosis and Fasting?

1. Take an intermittent fasting program – eat all meals (from breakfast to lunch, or from lunch to dinner) within an eight-hour time frame each day. Fast for the remaining 16 hours. If all of this is new to you and the idea of making changes in your diet and eating habits scares you too much, simply start by eating your usual meals during this time. Once it becomes a routine, continue implementing the ketogenic diet, and then making it cyclical. You can find comfort in knowing that once you reach the third step you can replenish some of your favorite healthy carbohydrates on a weekly basis.

If you want to maximize the health benefits of fasting further, consider switching to regular five-day fasting on water alone. For example, I do it three or four times a year. To simplify this process, gradually reach a point where you fast for twenty hours a day and eat two meals in just four hours. After a month, fasting while consuming only water for five days will not be that difficult.

2. Switch to a ketogenic diet until you generate measurable ketones – the three main stages are: limit the net carbohydrates (total carbohydrates without fiber) from 20 to 50 grams per day; replace the eliminated carbohydrates with healthy fats in order to obtain 50 to 85% of the daily caloric intake from fats and limit the protein to half a gram for every half kilo of lean body mass.

Avoid all trans fats and polyunsaturated vegetable oils that are not fine. Adding these harmful fats can cause more damage than excess carbohydrates, so just because a food is "high in fat" doesn't mean you should eat it. Keep these portions of net carbohydrates, fats and proteins until you get into ketosis and your body burns fat as an energy source. To determine that you are ketotic, you can use the ketone test strips, checking that the ketones in your blood are in the range of 0.5 to 3.0 mmol / L.

Remember that precision is important when it comes to portions of these nutrients. In fact, an excess of net carbohydrates will prevent ketosis as the body will first use any available glucose source, being a type of fuel that burns faster. Since it is practically impossible to determine the amount of fat accurately, net carbohydrates and proteins in all dishes, make sure you have some basic measuring and tracking tools at your fingertips.

3. Once you have verified you are in ketosis, start cycling in and out of ketosis by replenishing high amounts of net carbohydrates once or twice a week. As a general recommendation, the amount of net carbohydrates triples during the days you fill up on carbohydrates.

Remember that the body will again be able to effectively burn fat at any time after a couple of weeks or a few months. As already mentioned, entering and exiting cyclically from nutritional ketosis will maximize biological benefits of regeneration and renewal, while at the same time minimizing potential negative sides of continuous ketosis. At this point, even if high or low carbohydrates are given once or twice a week, I would still advise you to be careful about what is healthy and what is not.

Chapter 10: What to Eat and Not to Eat During Intermittent Fasting

No matter how you plot your path when it comes to an intermittent fast, you need to have an understanding of what is good to eat, and not to eat during your efforts. Unless you are engaging in a complete fast from solid foods for 24 hours, you will have to know just what you should eat on your fast days. Likewise, it would be good to know what might be best suited for your non-fast days too. Because remember, just because you might be on one of your non-fast days, doesn't mean it would be a good idea to go downtown and binge at all you can eat buffet. Here in this chapter, we will help guide you to make wise food choices on what to eat and what not to eat during your intermittent fasting.

What to Eat

Coffee

Okay, well it's not really a food, but coffee as a zero-calorie beverage is a great supplement to any fast day. Most of us can't do without a cup of coffee in the morning as it is, so this is most certainly good news for those of us who enjoy our cup of morning joe. Coffee can also help to ameliorate possible negative reactions to fasting. If your initial fast has you feeling a bit lethargic and lacking in energy, for example, a good stiff cup of coffee could certainly help to offset those symptoms. But keep in mind that the coffee needs to be taken straight out of the pot, foregoing any creams or sugars. For some of you, unsweetened coffee just might have to be an acquired taste, but if you ditch the sugars and creams, you will be a lot better off in the long run.

Raspberries

Raspberries are a low-calorie food that won't wreck your fast day and at the same time, will help keep you regular by giving you a healthy dose of fiber. Raspberries also come replete with healthy vitamins and minerals, as well as inflammation-busting antioxidants. This is good to ward off arthritis and other degenerative conditions. In some situations, raspberries are even said to prevent cancer. This is due to the powerful cancer-busting phytochemicals it boasts, called "ellagic acid." At any rate, if you have nothing else to eat on a fast day, a bowl of plain, simple, raspberries would be a good dietary choice to make.

Low-Calorie Beans and Legumes

Beans, beans, the magical fruit. The more you eat, the more fat you can burn for your fast. Both beans and legumes are packed with healthy nutrients and are typically low in calories. They also have plenty of protein, helping to keep your muscles fueled even while your fat stores are depleted. Tiny but mighty, beans and legumes are fully capable of aiding in the process of weight reduction, during your intermittent fast. Most especially good when it comes to intermittent fasting are peas, black beans, lentils, and garbanzo beans.

Blueberries

These fruitful treats are low in calories yet high in antioxidants, helping to ensure the body remains free of nasty free radicals that could degrade bodily tissue over time. Blueberries are known immune boosters too, good for ensuring you don't get sick or otherwise compromised while you fast. Another neat thing about blueberries is that they contain a little something called flavonoids, which if consumed over a long period of time, can work to reduce overall BMI (Body Mass Index). This is most definitely a good thing. And did I mention? They also taste great!

Eggs

Whether you hard boil them, scramble them, or poach them—the incredible, edible egg is a great low calorie, nutrient-dense food for your fast days. Eggs just seem especially geared for this task. Eggs have a ton of proteins and tend to stick with you, leaving you feeling full and satisfied. If you are indeed allowing a small allotment of under 500 calories on your fast day, adding a couple of eggs to the mix certainly won't ruin your fast.

Lean Chicken Breast

If you aren't doing a 24 hour fast, a serving of lean chicken breast is a good way to end a fast day that shouldn't exceed your 500-calorie allotment. Lean chicken breast provides plenty of proteins without all the filler of other sides of the meat. It's also a mainstay that goes well with quite a few meals and recipes. Here, in this book for one, you will find plenty of dishes that make full use of the power of a piece of lean chicken. Having that said, you should definitely stock up on some lean chicken breast in preparation for your next intermittent fast.

Fish

Just like chicken, fish is a good source of protein and yet won't break your budget of allotted calories on your fast day. Fish has a ton of what are known as omega-3 fatty acids. Don't let the "fat" word scare you though because omega-3 fatty acids are a good thing. There's a reason why every health food store has aisle after aisle of omega-3 supplements. Because its omega-3 fatty acids can safeguard our heart, dramatically reduce blood pressure, clear out plaque from arteries, and even prevent heart attacks and strokes. Fish is also considered a "brain food" due to its ability to help enhance cognitive function. Fish—it's decidedly nutritious, and it's downright delicious! Be sure to make use of it.

Veggies

You don't have to be a vegetarian to appreciate the tremendous benefit that veggies can provide. Vegetables represent a stabilizing force on your non-fast day and every day between. As well as providing plenty of valuable nutrients, veggies also give us a healthy dose of fiber to help keep us regular. Vegetables are typically low in calories too, so you can mix and match them with all kinds of meals regardless of meal plans. Be sure to have plenty of fresh veggies on hand.

Whole Grains

Whole grains are a great source of nutrition on fast or non-fast day either one. Unlike refined grains that spike your insulin, these morsels won't make you mess up your fast, and will still leave you feeling full and satisfied. You will find quite a few recipes in this book that make use of whole grain. It makes for a good bread alternative, so if you are ever in doubt—just reach for the whole grains!

Yogurt

When people think of healthy foods, one of the first things that come to mind is probably yogurt. Yogurt is an excellent source of nutrients and also provides a boost to your metabolism and energy even as you fast. Yogurts also come complete with a dose of probiotics that once ingested will work around the clock to keep your gut in good shape. The experts are stressing more and more that so-called good gut bacteria is the key to good health. Having that said, yogurt is a safe way to get plenty of it. Yogurt certainly does help when it comes to your preparation for your intermittent fasting regimen.

Dark Chocolate

I know not everyone is a fan of dark chocolate, and perhaps it's an acquired taste. But whether it takes you a while to appreciate it or not, the health benefits are immediate. Dark chocolate gives you a boost of energy even while fortifying your system with valuable antioxidants. The kind of antioxidants capable of fighting off cancer no less. Simply put, dark chocolate is some powerful stuff. With so much going for it, dark chocolate is a go-to food when it comes to intermittent fasting.

Coconut Oil

Coconut oil is a low-calorie, known metabolism booster, and will get your system up and running during your period of intermittent fasting. Coconut oil is good because it doesn't trigger insulin production unlike other oils do. You can use coconut oil as a supplement, or even a cooking aid, without any fear of disrupting your fast in the process. It's really quite a wonderful ingredient and you will see it made use of quite extensively in the recipes in this book.

What Not to Eat

Soda

What no soda? You've got to be kidding me! Sorry folks, I like a good fountain drink of soda just like the next person, but I'm afraid it's all too true. If you want to engage in intermittent fasting, you are going to have to leave your soda behind. This is not meant as a punishment—it's simply the reality of the beast. One of the major components of an intermittent fast, after all, is the avoidance of sugar. It's so your body will start burning fat stores already in place that during fasting we refrain from guzzling sugary soda for our metabolic rate to nibble on. So yes, for the time being, as you engage in an intermittent fasting routine, you will indeed have to forego soda.

Heavily Processed Food

As you have probably already picked up during the course of this book, processed foods are frowned upon. Anything that has been processed and packaged is going to have a ton of preservatives packed into them, that while generally harmless, will have a long-term effect on your system over time. Heavily processed food will also pose a direct interference with your metabolism. That's why the fresher the food, the better when it comes to intermittent fasting.

Sugary Sweets

Just like with sugary sodas, sugary sweets would be completely counterproductive for an intermittent fast. The goal of an intermittent fast after all is to switch the body from burning sugar and carbs, to burning our latent fat deposits instead. Eating sugary sweets would disrupt this process and instead just add more junk to the fat already deposited in our trunk. So yes, you must avoid sugary sweets at all costs while you participate in intermittent fasting.

Alcohol

I don't mean to be a party pooper or anything, but let me just go ahead and say it. Alcohol and intermittent fasting do not mix. The reason? Alcohol has a direct effect on fat-burning metabolism. And the last thing that you would want to do is wreck your fast by throwing a wrench in your fat-burning metabolism! Alcohol also carries, carbs, sugars, calories, and the like. So, yeah just like drinking and driving—drinking and fasting should be avoided.

Refined Grains

Unlike whole grains, refined grains will indeed have a decidedly negative impact on your fast. Refined grains once metabolized will actually turn directly into sugar. As already mentioned, a few times in this chapter, sugar will defeat the purpose of your fast. The whole purpose of intermittent fasting is to get your body to stop burning sugar as fuel and burn fat instead. Ingesting refined grains that turn into sugar, therefore, completely negates this process. It will also raise your insulin levels. Having that said, refined grains are to be avoided if at all possible.

Trans-Fat

To be perfectly blunt, trans-fats are just bad. No good can come from them. And most especially, no good could come from your fast by ingesting them. Trans-fat, the fatty acids found in certain milk and meat products should be avoided while you participate in an intermittent fast. It raises, cholesterol, insulin, and wrecks any chance you may have had of having a successful fast. Just say no, when it comes to trans-fat.

Fast Food

Even though we call it "fast food"—the burgers and fries we bag from places like McDonald's are not exactly the best thing to eat during an intermittent fast! One look at an overly processed, carb-dense meal from McDonald's and I think you might probably understand why.

At any rate, presented here are the foods that you should and shouldn't eat. Take note and take heart. Enjoy your fast!

Chapter 11: Weekly Meal Plan with Low-Carb and Keto Recipes

You can use the following meal plan below, but make sure to align it to the kind of plan you will implement, such as 16:8 or 5:2. If you are doing the 16:8 fasting plan, you can only consume the first half of the meals because you will need to set a window of 8 hours per day for food consumption while the remaining hours are devoted to fasting. You can eat the meals from breakfast up to lunch or lunch to evening or either of the two. Just make sure that it is in the eight-hour time frame.

On the other hand, if you are doing a 5:2 diet, what you should do is to omit two days from the meal plan (any day will do) as you need to eat normally for 5 days. The meals on the remaining two days should be modified by reducing your consumption so it will meet the 500 to 600 calories a day. If you are not currently fasting, you can use the meal plan as is without any modifications.

Day 1 (1316 Calories)

Breakfast: Deviled Eggs

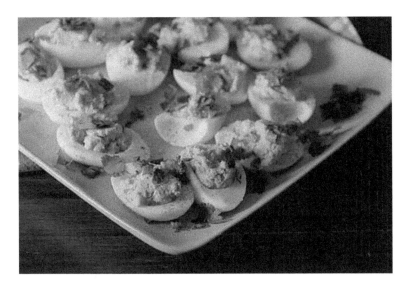

Cook Time: 20 minutes

Servings: 6

Ingredients:

- 8 oz. full-fat cream cheese, softened at room temperature

- 12 eggs

- 2 tablespoons everything bagel seasoning

- ½ teaspoon salt

- 1 grind black pepper

Instructions:

1. Add eggs to cold water, bring to a boil and cook for 10 minutes. Drain and add to cold water, let rest for 1-2 minutes. Peel the eggs.

2. Cut eggs in half lengthwise and scoop out the yolks. Add yolks to the bowl.

3. Slice cream cheese and add to the bowl with yolks. Blend well. Add in the salt and pepper and beat well.

4. Fill egg whites with the yolk mixture. Add seasoning son top. Serve.

Nutritional info (per serving): Calories 277; Total fat 22.6g; Saturated fat 10.5g; Protein 14.9g; Total carbs 3.3g; Net carbs 3.1g; Fiber 0.2g; Sugar 1.6 g

Lunch: Caesar Salad with Chicken

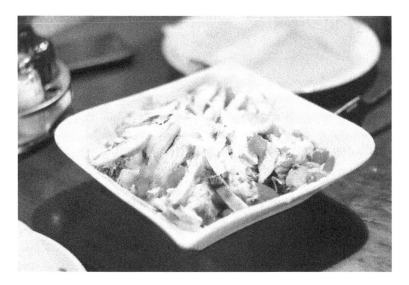

Cook Time: 15 minutes

Servings: 4

Ingredients:

- 2 chicken breasts, grilled

- 1 head Romaine lettuce, chopped

- 2 cup grape tomatoes, halved

- Parmesan cheese strips

For the Dressing:

- 3 garlic cloves, minced

- ½ lemon, juiced

- 1½ teaspoon Dijon mustard

- ¾ cup mayonnaise

- 1½ teaspoons anchovy paste

- 1 teaspoon Worcestershire sauce

- Salt and pepper, to taste

Instructions:

1. Mix all the dressing ingredients in a bowl and whisk well to combine. Cover and refrigerate the salad dressing.

2. Mix grape tomatoes, romaine lettuce, and cooked chicken in a bowl. Crumble the cheese crisps into smaller pieces. Add dressing on top.

3. Toss to combine and serve.

Nutritional info (per serving): Calories 400; Total fat 25g; Saturated fat 12g; Protein 33g; Total carbs 9g; Net carbs 5g; Fiber 4g; Sugar 4 g

Snack: Coconut Chocolate Chip Cookies

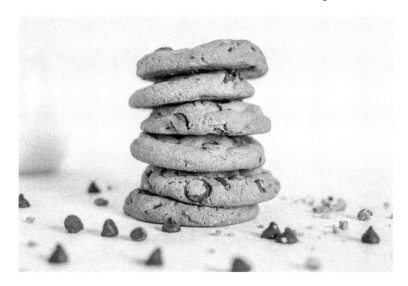

Cook Time: 30 minutes

Servings: 6

Ingredients:

- ¾ cup coconut, shredded

- 1¼ cups almond flour

- 1 teaspoon baking powder

- ½ cup butter (softened)

- ½ cup Swerve sweetener

- ½ teaspoon vanilla extract

- 1 egg

- ½ cup chocolate chips, sugar-free

- ½ teaspoon salt

Instructions:

1. Preheat the oven to 325°F and line a baking sheet with parchment paper.

2. Mix coconut, almond flour, baking powder, and salt in a bowl.

3. Mix butter with sweetener in a separate bowl. Beat in egg and vanilla. Stir to combine. Add this mixture to the flour mixture and beat it well. Add in the chocolate chips.

4. Shape the dough into 1½-inch balls. Place on the baking sheet 2 inches apart. Press each ball to ¼-inch thick.

5. Bake for 15 minutes. Remove from the oven and cool completely. Serve.

Nutritional info (per serving): Calories 268; Total fat 17.4g; Saturated fat 10.3g; Protein 12g; Total carbs 13g; Net carbs 12g; Fiber 1g; Sugar 10g

Dinner: Balsamic Chicken with Roasted Vegetables

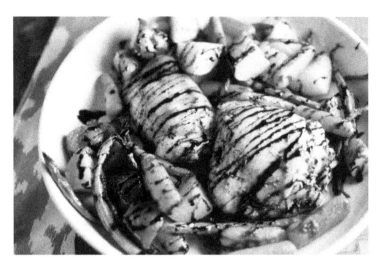

Cook Time: 30 minutes

Servings: 4

Ingredients:

- 10 asparaguses, ends trimmed and cut in half

- 8 boneless, skinless chicken thighs, fat trimmed

- 2 bell peppers, sliced into strips

- ½ cup carrots, sliced into half long and cut into 3-inch pieces

- 1 red onion, chopped into large chunks

- ¼ cup + 1 tablespoon balsamic vinegar

- 5 oz. mushrooms, sliced

- 2 tablespoons olive oil

- ½ tablespoon dried oregano

- 2 sage leaves, chopped

- 2 garlic cloves, smashed and chopped

- ½ teaspoon sugar

- 1½ tablespoons rosemary

- 1 teaspoon salt

- Black pepper, to taste

- Cooking spray

Instructions:

1. Preheat the oven to 425°F.

2. Season chicken with salt and pepper and spray 2 large baking sheets with cooking spray.

3. Mix all the ingredients in a bowl and mix well. Place everything on the prepared baking sheet and spread it in a single layer.

4. Bake for 25 minutes. Serve.

Nutritional info (per serving): Calories 450; Total fat 17g; Saturated fat 3g; Protein 48g; Total carbs 15g; Net carbs 4g; Fiber 11g; Sugar 2g

Day 2 (1358 Calories)

Breakfast: Cream Cheese Pancakes

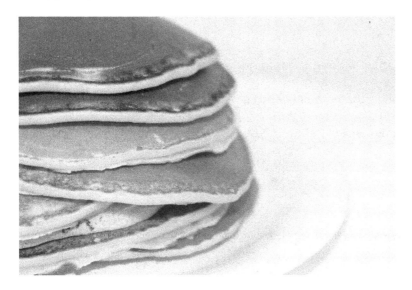

Cook Time: 15 minutes

Servings:

Ingredients:

- 2 eggs

- 4 oz. cream cheese

- ½ teaspoon baking powder

- ¼ cup almond flour

- ¼ teaspoon fine salt

- Cooking spray

- 3 tablespoons butter

Instructions:

1. Mix eggs, flour, cream cheese, baking powder, and salt in a blender and blend until smooth.

2. Heat a frying pan over medium heat and grease with cooking spray.

3. Add 3 tablespoons of butter. Cook for 3 minutes.

4. Flip and cook for 2 more minutes. Transfer to a plate.

5. Repeat with the remaining batter.

6. Serve.

Nutritional info (per serving): Calories 329; Total fat 30.2g; Saturated fat 16.7g; Protein 10.1g; Total carbs 5.4g; Net carbs 4.2g; Fiber 1.3g; Sugar 2.9g

Lunch: Thai Beef Salad

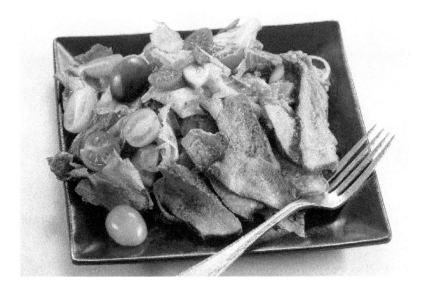

Cook Time: 15 minutes

Servings: 4

Ingredients:

- 1½ lb. flank steak

- 1 tablespoon olive oil

- 1 teaspoon sea salt

- 1 cup cucumbers, chopped

- 1 head lettuce, chopped

- 1 cup grape tomatoes, halved

- ¼ cup basil, cut into ribbons

- ¼ cup cilantro, chopped

- ¼ cup red onion, sliced

- ¼ cup olive oil

- ¼ cup coconut aminos

- 1 tablespoon fish sauce

- 2 tablespoon lime juice

- 1 tablespoon Thai red curry paste

Instructions:

1. Mix oil, coconut aminos, fish sauce, lime juice, and curry paste in a bowl and whisk to combine.

2. Season steak with salt on all sides. Put steak slices in a single layer into a glass baking dish. Add half of the marinade over the steak.

3. Cover meat with plastic wrap and refrigerate for 8 hours. Cover the reserved dressing and refrigerate.

4. Mix lettuce, cucumbers, grape tomatoes, cilantro, red onion, and basil in a bowl. Cook beef in a hot pan until brown on all sides. Let beef rest for 5 minutes. Slice against the grain.

5. Serve salad with beef and dressing.

Nutritional info (per serving): Calories 426; Total fat 26g; Saturated fat 14.2g; Protein 38g; Total carbs 8g; Net carbs 7g; Fiber 1g; Sugar 2g

Snack: Buffalo Chicken Sausage Balls

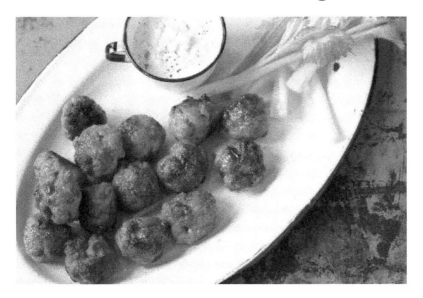

Cook Time: 40 minutes

Servings: 12 balls

Ingredients:

- 3 tablespoons coconut flour

- 24 oz. bulk chicken sausage

- 1 cup cheddar cheese, shredded

- 1 cup almond flour

- ½ cup Buffalo wing sauce

- ½ teaspoon cayenne

- 1 teaspoon salt

- ½ teaspoon pepper

- 2 garlic cloves, minced

- 1 teaspoon dried dill

- ⅓ cup mayonnaise

- ⅓ cup almond milk, unsweetened

- ½ teaspoon dried parsley

- ¼ cup bleu cheese, crumbled

- ½ teaspoon salt

- ½ teaspoon pepper

Instructions:

1. Preheat the oven to 350°F and line 2 baking sheets with parchment paper.

2. Mix cheddar cheese, sausage, almond flour, coconut flour, buffalo sauce, cayenne, salt, and pepper in a bowl and mix well until combined.

3. Roll the mixture into 1-inch balls and place on the baking sheets 1 inch apart. Bake for 25 minutes.

4. Mix mayo, almond milk, garlic, parsley, dill, salt, and pepper in a bowl. Mix well and add bleu cheese in. Mix well.

5. Serve balls with the sauce.

Nutritional info (per serving): Calories 255; Total fat 19.3g; Saturated fat 4.7g; Protein 15.3g; Total carbs 4.2g; Net carbs 2.5g; Fiber 1.7g; Sugar 5g

Dinner: Low Carb Chili

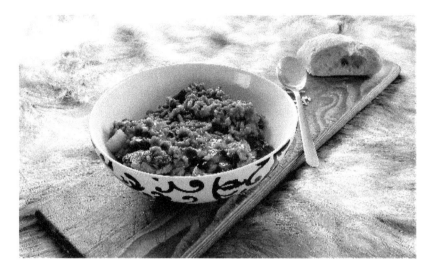

Cook Time: 40 minutes

Servings: 6

Ingredients:

- 1 bell pepper, chopped

- 1¼ lb. ground beef

- 8 oz. tomato paste

- 1½ tomato, chopped

- 2 celery sticks, chopped

- ½ cup onion, chopped

- 1½ teaspoons cumin

- ¾ cup of water

- 1½ teaspoon chili powder

- 1½ teaspoons salt

- ½ teaspoon pepper

Instructions:

1. Cook the meat in a frying pan until brown. Drain the excess fat and season meat with salt.

2. Add peppers and onions to the pan and cook for 2 minutes. Mix onions, cooked meat, peppers, tomatoes, water, celery, and tomato paste in a pot.

3. Add the spices to the pot. Bring to a boil and reduce the heat to low-medium. Cook for 2 hours while stirring every 30 minutes. Serve.

Nutritional info (per serving): Calories 348; Total fat 28.8g; Saturated fat 8.5g; Protein 14.9g; Total carbs 7.2g; Net carbs 5.2g; Fiber 2g; Sugar 3.3g

Day 3 (1471 Calories)

Breakfast: Oat-Free Porridge

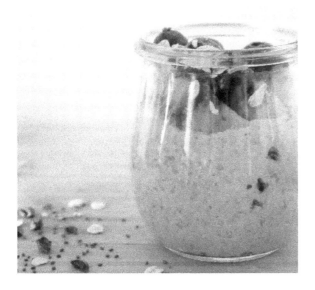

Cook Time: 5 minutes

Servings: 1

Ingredients:

- 2 tablespoons unsweetened coconut, shredded

- ½ cup of water

- 2 tablespoons hemp hearts

- 2 tablespoons almond flour

- 1 tablespoon chia seeds

- 1 tablespoon golden flaxseed meal

- ¼ teaspoon granulated stevia

- ½ teaspoon pure vanilla extract

- 1 pinch salt

Instructions:

1. Add all ingredients except vanilla to a saucepan.

2. Cook over low heat for 5 minutes, stirring constantly.

3. Add in the vanilla.

4. Serve.

Nutritional info (per serving): Calories 453; Total fat 36g; Saturated fat 10g; Protein 18g; Total carbs 15g; Net carbs 5g; Fiber 10g; Sugar 1g

Lunch: Caprese Zucchini Noodle Pasta Salad

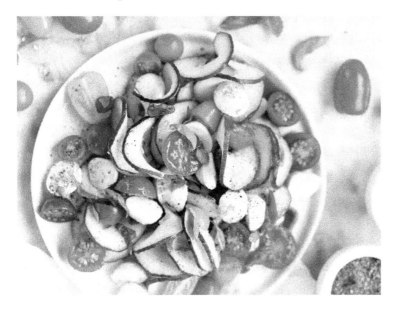

Cook Time: 15 minutes

Servings: 8 cups

Ingredients:

- 8 oz. mozzarella pearls

- 1 oz. basil, chopped

- 4 zucchinis, spiralized

- 4 oz. cherry tomatoes, sliced in half

- 3 tablespoon red wine vinegar

- ¼ cup extra virgin olive oil

- 1 tablespoon lemon juice

- ¼ teaspoon garlic powder

- ½ teaspoon salt

- ¼ teaspoon pepper

Instructions:

1. Whisk red wine, oil, lemon juice, garlic powder, salt, and pepper in a bowl.

2. Add the remaining ingredients to a bowl and add dressing on top.

3. Toss well to combine. Serve.

Nutritional info (per serving): Calories 186; Total fat 13g; Saturated fat 4g; Protein 7g; Total carbs 4g; Net carbs 3g; Fiber 1g; Sugar 3g

Snack: Bacon and Guacamole Fat Bombs

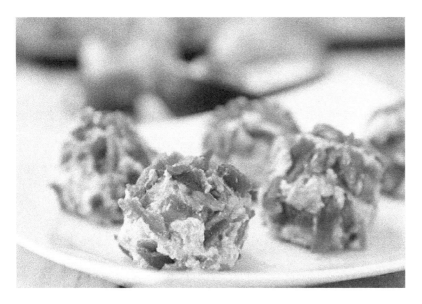

Cook Time: 45 minutes

Servings: 6

Ingredients:

- ¼ cup butter (softened)

- ½ avocado

- 2 garlic cloves, crushed

- ½ small white onion, diced

- 1 small chili pepper, finely chopped

- 1 tablespoon lime juice

- 2 tablespoons cilantro, chopped

- 4 slices bacon

- ¼ teaspoon sea salt

- Black pepper

Instructions:

1. Preheat the oven to 375°F and line a baking tray with baking paper. Place the bacon strips on the baking tray.

2. Bake for 15 minutes. Remove the tray from the oven and let cool. Crumble the bacon.

3. Cut avocado in half, remove the pit and peel it. Add butter, avocado, chili pepper, cilantro, crushed garlic, and lime juice to a bowl. Season with salt and pepper. Mash with a fork until combined.

4. Add onion and mix. Add bacon grease from the baking tray and mix well. Cover with foil and refrigerate for 30 minutes.

5. Shape the guacamole mixture into 6 balls. Roll each ball into the bacon pieces and place on a tray. Serve.

Nutritional info (per serving): Calories 156; Total fat 15.2g; Saturated fat 6.8g; Protein 3.4g; Total carbs 2.7g; Net carbs 1.4g; Fiber 1.3g; Sugar 0.5g

Dinner: Cheesy Tuna Pesto Pasta

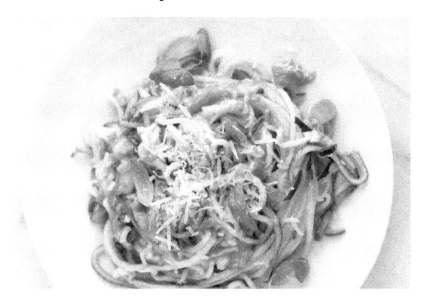

Cook Time: 25 minutes

Servings: 4

Ingredients:

- 4 cups zucchini noodles, spiralized, cooked

- 1 cup cheddar, grated

- 1 cup yellowfin tuna in olive oil

- 7 oz. basil pesto

- 1½ cup punnet cherry tomato, halved

Instructions:

1. Mix pesto and tuna with oil in a bowl. Mash well. Add in ⅓ of the cheese and add all the tomatoes.

2. Add noodles to the bowl, toss well to coat. Transfer the mixture to a baking dish and add the remaining cheese on top.

3. Broil the dish for 4 minutes. Serve.

Nutritional info (per serving): Calories 696; Total fat 27g; Saturated fat 11g; Protein 40g; Total carbs 14g; Net carbs 10g; Fiber 4g; Sugar 5g

Day 4 (1521 Calories)

Breakfast: Keto Breakfast Bowl

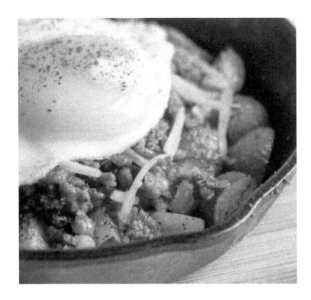

Cook Time: 30 minutes

Servings: 1

Ingredients:

- 1 egg

- ¼ cup cheddar cheese, shredded

- 2 cups radishes

- 3½ oz. ground sausage

- ¼ teaspoon pink Himalayan salt

- ¼ teaspoon black pepper

Instructions:

1. Cook sausage in a pan over medium-high heat until done. Remove sausage from the pan and set aside.

2. Cut radishes into small pieces and add to the pan. Season well. Cook radishes for 12 minutes.

3. Fry the egg the way you want and set aside.

4. Layer the radishes with sausage on a plate, top with egg and cheese.

5. Serve.

Nutritional info (per serving): Calories 617; Total fat 49g; Saturated fat 11.1g; Protein 32g; Total carbs 7g; Net carbs 4g; Fiber 3g; Sugar 5g

Lunch: Kale and Brussels Sprout Salad

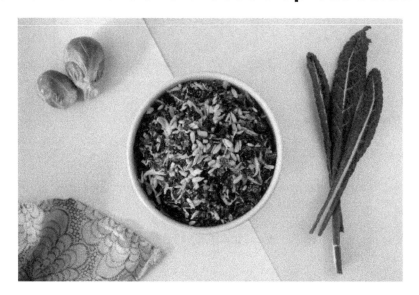

Cook Time: 15 minutes

Servings: 8

Ingredients:

- ½ lb. Brussels sprouts, outer leaves, and stems removed

- ½ bunch curly kale

- 6 slices cooked bacon

- ½ cup dried cranberries

- ½ cup walnuts

- 2 tablespoons lemon juice

- ⅓ cup olive oil

- ½ teaspoon garlic powder

- 1 tablespoon Dijon mustard

- ¼ teaspoon sea salt

- ¼ teaspoon black pepper

Instructions:

1. Add Brussels sprouts to a blender and blend well until chopped.

2. Add kale leaves to it and pulse until shredded.

3. Whisk mustard, olive oil, lemon juice, garlic powder, salt, and pepper in a bowl until well mixed.

4. Add kale and Brussels sprouts and stir to combine. Add the cooked bacon, walnuts, and cranberries in it. Toss well. Serve.

Nutritional info (per serving): Calories 192; Total fat 17g; Saturated fat 1.6g; Protein 6g; Total carbs 6g; Net carbs 4g; Fiber 2g; Sugar 3g

Snack: Cheddar Jalapeno Meatballs

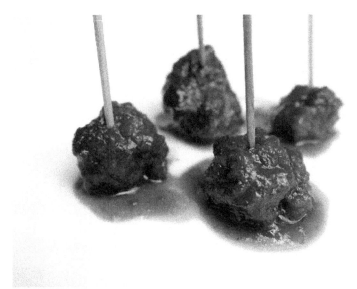

Cook Time: 45 minutes

Servings: 8

Ingredients:

- 1½ lb. ground beef

- 1 large jalapeno, sliced

- 6 oz. sharp cheddar, grated

- ½ cup pork rind crumbs

- 1 egg

- 1 teaspoon chili powder

- 2 tablespoons cilantro, chopped

- 1 teaspoon garlic powder

- ½ teaspoon cumin

- 1 teaspoon salt

- ½ teaspoon pepper

Instructions:

1. Preheat the oven to 375°F and line a rimmed baking sheet with parchment paper.

2. Mix all ingredients in a blender. Blend on high until well combined. Roll the dough into 1½-inch balls and add to the baking sheet 1 inch apart.

3. Bake for 20 minutes.

4. Serve.

Nutritional info (per serving): Calories 368; Total fat 24g; Saturated fat 9.7g; Protein 33.4g; Total carbs 1.1g; Net carbs 0.8g; Fiber 0.3g; Sugar 1g

Dinner: Keto Meatloaf

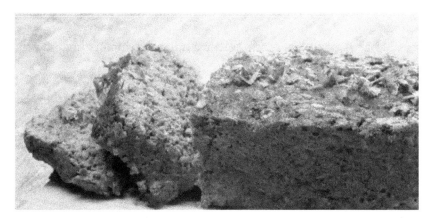

Cook Time: 1 hour

Servings: 6

Ingredients:

- 2 eggs

- 2 lbs. 85% lean grass-fed ground beef

- ¼ cup nutritional yeast

- 1 tablespoon lemon zest

- 2 tablespoons avocado oil

- ¼ cup parsley, chopped

- 4 garlic cloves

- ¼ cup oregano, chopped

- ½ tablespoon pink Himalayan salt

- 1 teaspoon black pepper

Instructions:

1. Preheat the oven to 400°F. Mix beef, yeast, salt, and pepper in a bowl.

2. Mix eggs, oil, garlic, and herbs in a blender and blend until everything is mixed well. Add this mixture to the beef and mix well.

3. Add the beef mixture to a small loaf pan. Arrange the pan on the middle rack and bake for 1 hour. Remove the pan from the oven. Let cool for 10 minutes.

4. Serve.

Nutritional info (per serving): Calories 344; Total fat 29g; Saturated fat 13.4g; Protein 33g; Total carbs 4g; Net carbs 2g; Fiber 2g; Sugar 1g

Day 5 (1371 Calories)

Breakfast: Sausage and Peppers No Egg Breakfast Bake

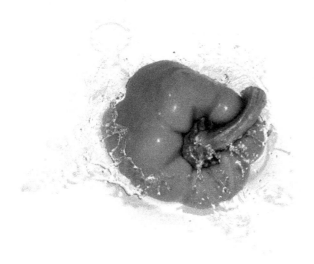

Cook Time: 50 minutes

Servings: 4

Ingredients:

- 1½ teaspoon olive oil

- 1 green bell pepper, chopped

- 1 red bell pepper, chopped

- ½ cup mozzarella cheese, grated

- 10 oz. sausage

- Salt, black pepper, to taste

Instructions:

1. Preheat the oven to 450°F and grease a medium-sized dish with cooking spray.

2. Add peppers to the baking dish and toss with 1 teaspoon olive oil and add salt and black pepper on top. Bake for 20 minutes.

3. Heat remaining olive oil on a pan and add the sausages. Cook over medium-high heat for 12 minutes.

4. Cut sausages into pieces. Add the sausages to the baking pan with the peppers. Bake for 5 more minutes.

5. Remove the dish from the oven, turn the oven to broil. Add the mozzarella over the peppers and sausages. Broil for 2 minutes. Serve.

Nutritional info (per serving): Calories 246; Total fat 13g; Saturated fat 5g; Protein 26g; Total carbs 5g; Net carbs 4g; Fiber 1g; Sugar 2g

Lunch: Curried Cabbage Coconut Salad

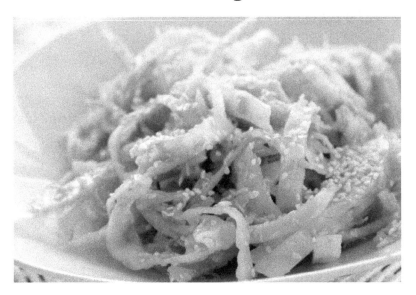

Cook Time: 5 minutes

Servings: 4

Ingredients:

- ¼ cup of coconut oil

- ½ head white cabbage, shredded

- 1 lemon juice

- ⅓ cup dried coconut, unsweetened

- ¼ cup tamari sauce

- ½ teaspoon ginger, dried

- 3 teaspoons sesame seeds

- ½ teaspoon curry powder

- ½ teaspoon cumin

Instructions:

1. Add all the ingredients to a bowl and toss well.

2. Cover and refrigerate for 1 hour. Serve.

Nutritional info (per serving): Calories 309; Total fat 5g; Saturated fat 8g; Protein 12g; Total carbs 12g; Net carbs 6g; Fiber 6g; Sugar 3g

Snack: Cheesy Party Crackers

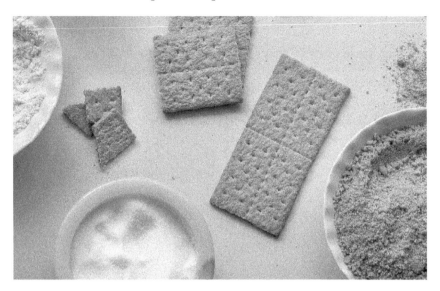

Cook Time: 45 minutes

Servings: 8

Ingredients:

- ½ cup flax meal

- 1 cup almond flour

- 2 tablespoons whole psyllium husks

- 1 cup of water

- 1 cup Parmesan cheese, grated

- 1 teaspoon salt

- ¼ teaspoon black pepper

Instructions:

1. Mix flax meal, almond flour, psyllium, salt, and pepper in a bowl.

2. Add the cheese to it and mix well. Add water and mix well. Let rest for 15 minutes.

3. Preheat the oven to 320°F and divide the dough into 2 parts.

Place half of the dough on a parchment paper. Place another piece of parchment paper on top and roll the dough out until thin.

4. Cut the dough into 16 equal pieces. Repeat the process with the remaining dough.

5. Bake for 45 minutes.

6. Serve.

Nutritional info (per serving): Calories 169; Total fat 13.4g; Saturated fat 2.7g; Protein 8.4g; Total carbs 6.3g; Net carbs 1.7g; Fiber 4.5g; Sugar 0.8 g

Dinner: Crispy Salmon with Pesto Cauliflower Rice

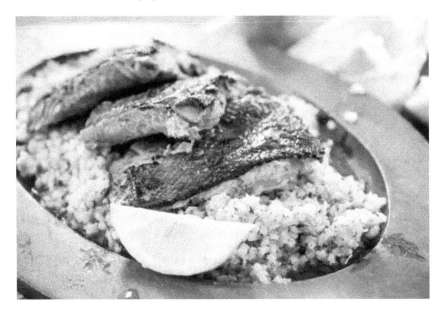

Cook Time: 40 minutes

Servings: 3

Ingredients:

- 1 tablespoon olive oil

- 3 salmon fillets

- 1 tablespoon coconut aminos

- 1 teaspoon fish sauce

- 1 tablespoon butter

- 3 garlic cloves

- 1 cup basil leaves, chopped

- ¼ cup hemp hearts

- ½ cup olive oil

- 1 lemon juice

- ½ teaspoon pink salt

- 3 cups riced cauliflower, frozen

- 1 scoop MCT Powder

- Pinch salt

Instructions:

1. Add fish sauce, coconut aminos, and olive oil to a baking dish. Pat the salmon fillets dry and add place into the dish skin side down. Add a pinch of salt. Let rest for 20 minutes.

2. Heat an iron skillet on medium heat.

3. Peel and dice the garlic and add it to a blender. Add hemp hearts, basil, lemon juice, olive oil, MCT powder, and salt. Pulse well to combine.

4. Heat cauliflower rice in a skillet. Add pesto and pink salt. Mix well to combine. Lower the heat and keep it warm.

5. Add butter to the iron skillet placed over medium heat. Add salmon skin side down. Cook for 5 minutes. Flip the salmon and add the remaining marinade from the plate. Sear for 2 minutes.

6. Remove from heat and serve on top of rice.

7. Enjoy!

Nutritional info (per serving): Calories 647; Total fat 51g; Saturated fat 10.8g; Protein 33.8g; Total carbs 8g; Net carbs 5g; Fiber 3g; Sugar 3g

Day 6 (1237 Calories)

Breakfast: Bacon and Egg Breakfast Muffins

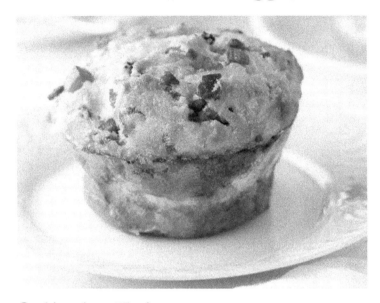

Cooking time: 25 minutes

Servings: 12

Ingredients:

- 8 eggs

- 8 bacon slices

- ⅔ cup green onion, chopped

- Cooking spray

Instructions:

1. Coat the muffin tin with nonstick cooking spray and preheat the oven to 350°F.

2. Add bacon to a large pan and cook over medium heat until crisp. Transfer to a plate lined with paper towels. Let cool and then chop into small pieces.

3. Add eggs to a bowl and whisk well. Then add green onions and cooked bacon. Mix until everything is well-combined.

4. Add the mixture to the muffin tin. Bake for about 20–25 minutes, until edges are golden brown.

5. Let the muffins cool and enjoy bacon and egg breakfast muffins.

Nutritional info (per serving): Calories 158; Total fat 13.3g; Saturated fat 1.7g; Protein 8g; Total carbs 1g; Net carbs 1g; Fiber 0g; Sugar 1g

Lunch: Grilled Chicken Salad

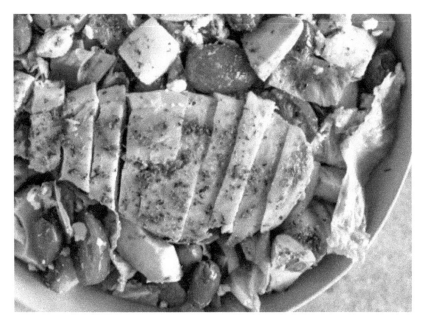

Cooking time: 20 minutes

Servings: 2

Ingredients:

- ½ lb. chicken thigh, grilled and sliced

- 1 teaspoon fresh thyme

- 4 cups romaine lettuce, chopped

- 2 garlic cloves, crushed

- ¼ cup cherry tomatoes, chopped

- 3 tablespoons extra virgin olive oil

- ½ cucumber, thinly sliced

- 2 tablespoons red wine vinegar

- ½ avocado, sliced

- 1 oz. olives, pitted and sliced

- 1 oz. Feta cheese, crumbled

- Salt, pepper, to taste

Instructions:

1. Season chicken with a teaspoon of thyme, crushed garlic, pepper, and salt.

2. Preheat oil in a pan over medium heat. Cook chicken until golden brown.

3. Mix olives, sliced cucumber, chopped lettuce, sliced avocado, and ¼ cup tomatoes in a large bowl.

4. Add chicken to the salad. Sprinkle with crumbled cheese.

5. Drizzle with olive oil and vinegar. Enjoy!

Nutritional info (per serving): Calories 617; Total fat 52g; Saturated fat 4g; Protein 30g; Total carbs 11g; Net carbs 7g; Fiber 4g; Sugar 2.5g

Snack: Keto Almond Bark

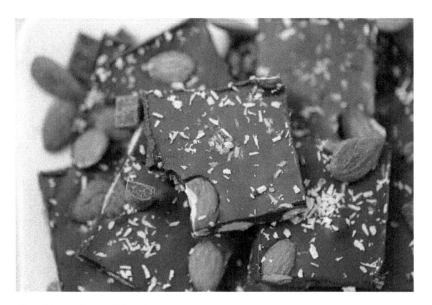

Cooking time: 15 minutes

Servings: 20

Ingredients:

- 4 oz. cocoa butter

- ½ cup Swerve sweetener

- ½ teaspoon vanilla extract

- 2 tablespoons water

- ¾ cup cocoa powder

- 1 tablespoon butter

- ½ cup powdered Swerve sweetener

- 1½ cups roasted almonds, unsalted

- 2½ oz. unsweetened chocolate, chopped

- ¼ teaspoon sea salt

Instructions:

1. Add 2 tablespoons of water and ½ cup Swerve sweetener to a saucepan. Bring the mixture to a light boil, stirring occasionally. Cook for about 8 to 9 minutes until the mixture darkens.

2. Turn the heat off and whisk in 1 tablespoon butter. Add 1½ cups roasted almonds and toss well until coated. Then stir in 2 pinches of salt.

3. Spread almonds onto a parchment-lined baking sheet. Add 4 oz. cocoa butter and 2½ oz. unsweetened chocolate to a large saucepan. Melt over medium heat and stir until smooth.

4. Stir in ¾ cup cocoa powder and ½ cup powdered Swerve sweetener until smooth. Turn the heat off and stir in ½ teaspoon vanilla extract.

5. Reserve 4 tablespoons of almonds and keep them aside. Add leftover almonds to the chocolate mixture and stir well.

6. Spread chocolate-almond mixture out onto the same baking sheet. Top with reserved ¼ cups of almonds and sprinkle with salt.

7. Chill for about 3 hours and then break into chunks. Serve right away!

Nutritional info (per serving): Calories 144; Total fat 14g; Saturated fat 1.3g; Protein 13g; Total carbs 5g; Net carbs 2g; Fiber 3g; Sugar 10 g

Dinner: Chicken Parmesan

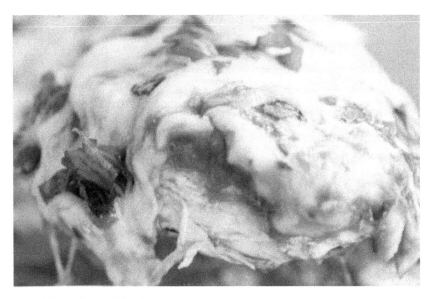

Cooking time: 19 minutes

Servings: 8

Ingredients:

- 2 lbs. boneless skinless chicken breast

- 4 oz. fresh mozzarella

- ⅓ cup sugar-free marinara

- 1 cup almond flour

- 1 cup parmesan cheese, grated

- 2 eggs

- 1 teaspoon Italian seasoning

- ½ teaspoon black pepper

- ½ teaspoon sea salt

Instructions:

1. Add chicken to a plastic bag and pound until about ½-inch thick.

2. Add 1 teaspoon Italian seasoning, a cup of parmesan cheese, ½ teaspoon sea salt, a cup of almond flour, and ½ teaspoon pepper. Mix well.

3. Add eggs to a separate bowl and whisk well. Pat dry the chicken with paper towels.

4. Dip chicken into the egg mixture and then coat with almond flour mixture. Brush with oil or coat with cooking spray.

5. Preheat the oven to 425°F. Place chicken on a baking sheet lined with parchment paper. Cook for about 11-12 minutes.

6. Then flip the chicken, spray with cooking spray and cook for 5 minutes more.

7. Sprinkle each piece with mozzarella and drizzle with pasta sauce. Transfer back to the oven and cook for a few minutes until cheese is melted.

Nutritional info (per serving): Calories 318; Total fat 17g; Saturated fat 5g; Protein 36g; Total carbs 4g; Net carbs 3g; Fiber 1g; Sugar 1g

Day 7 (1258 Calories)

Breakfast: Chocolate Mint Avocado Smoothie

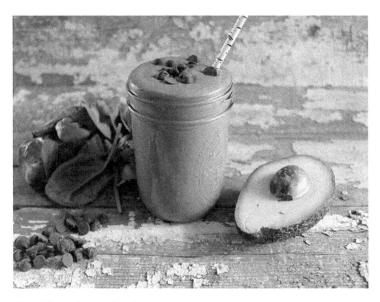

Cooking time: 5 minutes

Servings: 1

Ingredients:

- 2 scoops of chocolate collagen protein

- 2 tablespoons coconut, shredded

- ½ cup of coconut milk

- 1 tablespoon cacao butter, crushed

- 1 cup of water

- 4 mint leaves

- ½ cup ice

- ½ a frozen avocado

Instructions:

1. Add all the ingredients except for shredded coconut and collagen protein to a blender.

2. Blend on high for about 45 seconds. Then add collagen protein to a blender and blend for 5 seconds more.

3. Top chocolate mint avocado smoothie with coconut flakes. Enjoy!

Nutritional info (per serving): Calories 552; Total fat 44g; Saturated fat 25g; Protein 26g; Total carbs 10g; Net carbs 1g; Fiber 9g; Sugar 2g

Lunch: Italian Salad

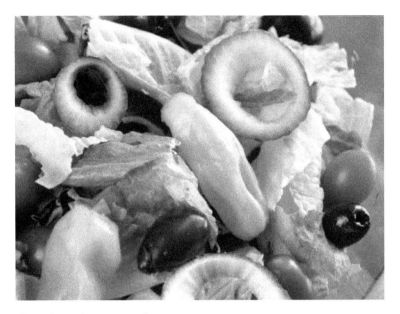

Cooking time: 15 minutes

Servings: 4

Ingredients:

- 1 cup mixed Italian olives, pitted

- 6 oz. deli ham, diced

- 6 cups Romaine lettuce, shredded

- ¼ cup pickled banana peppers, sliced

- 2 medium Roma tomatoes, diced

- ¼ red onion, sliced

For the Vinaigrette:

- 1 tablespoon red wine vinegar

- 1 tablespoon Italian seasoning

- ½ cup olive oil

- A pinch of sea salt

- Black pepper, to taste

Instructions:

1. Add all vinaigrette ingredients to a bowl and whisk well to combine.

2. Arrange all the salad ingredients in a large bowl and top with the dressing. Toss well to combine.

3. Enjoy!

Nutritional info (per serving): Calories 289; Total fat 24g; Saturated fat 7g; Protein 11g; Total carbs 7g; Net carbs 4g; Fiber 3g; Sugar 3g

Snack: Brussels Sprouts Chips

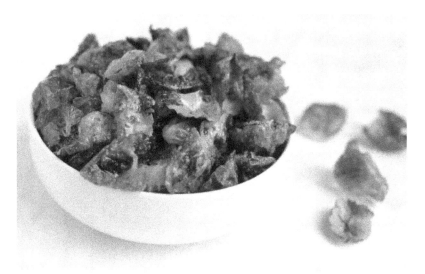

Cooking time: 15-20 minutes

Servings: 4

Ingredients:

- 1 lb. Brussels sprouts washed and dried, ends trimmed

- 1 teaspoon salt

- 2 tablespoons extra virgin olive oil

- Smoked paprika, for serving

Instructions:

1. Preheat the oven to 400°F

2. Peel the outer leaves of the Brussels sprouts and discard them. Add the sprouts to a bowl.

3. Drizzle with oil and toss well to coat in oil. Season with salt. Spread on a baking sheet evenly in one layer.

4. Bake for about 12–15 minutes. Take them out from the oven and let them cool.

5. Sprinkle with more salt if you want. Serve topped with smoked paprika.

Nutritional info (per serving): Calories 104; Total fat 7g; Saturated fat 1.4g; Protein 3g; Total carbs 9g; Net carbs 5g; Fiber 4g; Sugar 1g

Dinner: Mushroom Bacon Skillet

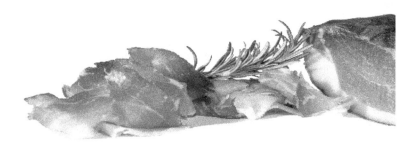

Cooking time: 10 minutes

Servings: 1

Ingredients:

- ½ teaspoon salt

- 1 tablespoon garlic, minced

- 4 slices pastured pork bacon, cut into ½-inch pieces

- 2 sprigs thyme, leaves only

- 2 cups mushrooms, halved

Instructions:

1. Preheat a skillet over medium heat. Add bacon and cook until crispy. Remove from the pan.

2. Add sliced mushrooms. Saute until soften, stirring often.

3. Add garlic, thyme, and salt. Cook for 5 minutes more, stirring often.

4. When mushrooms become golden, turn the heat off.

5. Garnish mushroom bacon with greens and enjoy!

Nutritional info (per serving): Calories 313; Total fat 8.5g; Saturated fat 3.8g; Protein 13.6g; Total carbs 8.4g; Net carbs 0.3g; Fiber 8.1g; Sugar 2.2g

Chapter 12: Possible Side Effects of The Diet

Even though we can't overlook the way that irregular fasting has a lot of medical advantages. The earlier mentioned are only a couple of them. There are significantly more favorable circumstances that are extraordinary for the human body and increment the life expectancy of people too. There are likewise some negative effects of intermittent fasting. Any individual who is going to begin irregular fasting at any point shortly has to know both the positive and negative effects of fasting and afterward choose either it's advantageous for your body or not.

Anxiety Attacks

Another potential side effect of detoxing through intermittent fasting is the potential for an anxiety attack. This can happen when you are withholding food for an extended period of time especially if you are new to intermittent fasting.

An anxiety attack may arise because you feel you are not eating enough, or because you are not keeping to your usual eating schedules.

Digestive Distress

Since intermittent fasting has a detoxing component to it, you may experience digestive distress during your first few experiences. This is due to your body flushing out much of the residual matter in your body in addition to simply excreting whatever is still leftover in the digestive tract.

While this is normal to a certain extent, care should be taken if you happen to experience severe diarrhea. This may be especially true if you jump into a fasting period after overeating the previous day. As long as it isn't anything that you feel to be abnormal, then you can attribute it to the detoxing process. However, if symptoms do not subside then you may need to seek medical attention at once.

You Might Struggle to Maintain Blood Sugar Levels

Although the intermittent fasting diet tends to improve blood sugar levels in most people, this is not always true for everyone. Some people who are eating following the intermittent fasting diet may find that their ability to maintain a healthy blood sugar level is compromised.

The reason why this happens varies. For some people, not eating frequently enough may encourage this to happen. For others, transitioning too quickly or taking on too intense of a fasting cycle too soon can result in a shock to the body that causes a strange fluctuation in blood sugar levels.

You Might Experience Hormonal Imbalances

A certain degree of fasting, especially when you build up to it, can support you in having healthier hormone levels. However, for some people, intermittent fasting may lead to an unhealthy imbalance of hormones. This can result in a whole slew of different hormone-based symptoms, such as headaches, fatigue, and even menstrual problems in women.

Again, the reason for the hormonal imbalance varies. For some people, particularly those who are already at risk of experiencing hormonal imbalances, intermittent fasting can trigger these imbalances to take place. For others, it could go back to what they are consuming during the eating windows. Eating meals that are not rich in nutrients and vitamins can result in you not having enough nutrition to support your hormonal levels.

If you begin experiencing hormonal imbalances when you eat the intermittent fasting diet, it is essential that you stop and consult your doctor right away. Discovering where the shortcomings are and how you can correct them is vital. Having imbalanced hormones for too long can lead to diseases and illnesses that require constant life-long attention.

Headaches

A decrease in your blood sugar level and the release of stress hormones by your brain as a result of going without food are possible causes of headaches during the fasting window. Problems may also be a clear message from your body telling you that you are very low on water and getting dehydrated. This may happen if you are completely engrossed in your daily activities, and you forget to drink the required amount of water your body needs during fasting.

To handle headaches, ensure you stay well hydrated throughout your fasting window. Keep in mind that exceeding the required amount of water per day may also result in adverse effects. Reducing your stress level can also keep headaches away.

Cravings

During your fasting periods, you might find that you have higher levels of desires than usual. This often happens because you are telling yourself that you cannot have any food, so suddenly you start craving many different foods. This is because all you are thinking about is food. As you think about food, you will begin to think about the different types of food that you like and that you want. Then, the cravings start.

Early on, you may also find yourself craving more sweets or carbs because your body is searching for an energy hit through glucose. While you do not want to have excessive levels of sugar during your eating window, as this is bad for blood sugar, you can always have some. The ability to satisfy your cravings is one of the benefits of eating a diet that is not as restrictive as some other foods are.

Low Energy

A feeling of lethargy is not uncommon during fasting, especially at the start. This is your body's natural reaction to switching its source of energy from glucose in your meals to fat stored in your body. So, expect to feel a little less energized in your first few weeks of starting with intermittent fasting. To troubleshoot the feeling of lethargy, try as much as possible to stay away from overly strenuous activities. Keep things low-key. Spending more time sleeping or just relaxing is another right way to ensure that your energy reserves are not depleted too quickly. The first few weeks are not the time to test your limits or push yourself.

Foul Mood

You may find yourself being on edge during fasting, even if you are someone who is naturally predisposed to being good-natured. The reason for the feeling of edginess is straightforward. You are hungry, yet you won't eat, and you are struggling to keep your cravings in check, plus, you may already be feeling tired and sluggish. Add all of these to the internal hormone changes due to the sharp decline in your blood sugar levels, and it's no wonder why you may be in such a foul mood. Tempers can easily flare up, and you may be quick to become irritated. This is normal when beginning a fasting lifestyle.

Excess Urination

Fasting tends to make you visit the bathroom more frequently than usual. This is an expected side effect since you are drinking more water and other liquids than before. Avoiding water to reduce the number of times you use the bathroom is not a good idea at all, no matter how you look at it. Cutting down water intake while you are fasting will make your body become dehydrated very quickly. If that happens, losing weight will be the least of your problems. Whatever you do, do not avoid drinking water when you are fasting. Doing that is paving the way for a humongous health disaster waiting to happen. You don't want to do that.

Heartburn, Bloating, and Constipation

Your stomach is responsible for producing stomach acid, which is used to break down food and trigger the digestion process. When you eat frequent meals, unusually large meals, regularly, your body is used to producing high amounts of stomach acid to break down your food. As you transition to a fasting diet, your stomach has to get used to not producing as much stomach acid.

You might also notice an increase in constipation and bloating. People who eat regularly consume high amounts of fiber and proteins that support a healthy digestion process. When you switch to the intermittent fasting cycle, you can still eat a high volume of fiber and protein. However, early on, you might find that you forget to. As you discover the right eating habits that work for you, it may take some time for you to get used to finding ways to work in enough fiber and protein to keep your digestion flowing.

Heartburn may not be a widespread adverse effect, but it does sometimes occur in some individuals. Your stomach produces highly concentrated acids to help break down the foods you consume. But when you are fasting, there is no food in your stomach to be broken down, even though acids have already been produced for that purpose. This may lead to heartburn.

Bloating and constipation usually go hand in hand and can be very discomforting to individuals who suffer from it due to fasting.

Heeding the advice to drink adequate amounts of water usually keeps bloating and constipation in check. Heartburn typically resolves itself quickly, but you can take an antacid tablet or two if it persists. You may also consider eating fewer spicy foods when you break your fast.

You Might Experience Low Energy and Irritability

Until now, your body has been used to having a constant stream of energy pouring in all day long. From the time you wake up until the time you go to bed, it has been receiving some form of power from the foods that you eat. So, when you stop eating regularly, your body grows confused. It has to learn to create its energy rather than rely on the heat being offered to it by the food that you are eating.

Depending on how you are eating, your body may also be growing used to consuming fat as a fuel source rather than carbohydrates. This means that, in addition to losing its primary energy source, it also has to switch how it consumes energy and where it comes from. This can lead to lowered energy for a while. Do things that exert the least amount of energy. If you are someone who regularly exercises and works out, reducing the amount that you work out or switching to a more relaxed workout like yoga can help you during the transition period.

You Might Start Feeling Cold

As you begin to adjust to your intermittent fasting diet, you might find that your fingers and toes get quite cold. This happens because blood flow towards your fat stores is increasing, so blood flow to your extremities reduces slightly. This supports your body in moving fat to your muscles so that it can be burned as fuel to keep your energy levels up.

You Might Find Yourself Overeating

The chances for overeating during the break of the fast are high, especially for beginners. Understandably, you will feel starving after going without food for longer than you are used to. It is this hunger that causes some people to eat hurriedly and surpass their standard meal size and average caloric intake. For others, overeating may be a result of an uncontrollable appetite. Hunger may push some people to prepare too much food for breaking their fast, and if they don't have a grip on their desire, they will continue to eat even when they are satiated. Overeating or binging when you break your fast will make it difficult to reach your goal of optimal health and fitness.

Hunger Pangs

People who start intermittent fasting may initially feel quite hungry. This is especially common if you are the type of person who tends to eat regular meals daily.

If you start feeling hungry, you can choose to wait it out if you have an eating window right around the corner. However, if there is a more extended waiting period or you are feeling excessively hungry, you should eat. Feeling hungry to the point that it becomes uncomfortable or distracting is not helpful and will not support you in successfully taking on the intermittent fasting diet. This is a pronounced side effect of going without food for longer than you are accustomed to.

Headaches

One other symptom that may affect you during fasting is a headache. This is a natural reaction by the brain to the sudden change in chemical composition as a result of the detoxing process. You may find that you get a slight headache, which will go away on its own.

However, a strong headache and persistent headache may be a side effect of the detoxing process or just a lack of food. Since you have an empty stomach, taking headache medication would be ill-advised as it may trigger digestive distress. If your headache is unbearable, then you may need to have food with the medication.

Chapter 13: Tips and Tricks to Start and Follow The IF

Intermittent fasting is not easy. We need support as much as possible and anything that can make your journey easier. Below are some of the tips that will make your journey smooth and effective.

Decide on your fasting window

Intermittent fasting is not a strict time-based diet. This means that you can choose the number of hours to fast and when to fast either day or night. The fasting and eating window periods are not a must to be the same every day.

Ensure you get enough sleep

When you get enough sleep, you become healthier, and your overall well-being is guaranteed. When we sleep, the body operates certain functions in the body that helps burn calories and improves the metabolic rate.

Eat healthy Avoid eating anything you want after a fast

Healthy meals should be your focus. They will help you get the required nutrients like vitamins, which will give you more energy during the fasting period.

Drink more water

One of the best decisions you can make during a fast is to drink water. It will keep your body hydrated and taking water before meals can significantly reduce appetite.

Start small

If you have never tried it before, there is no way you start fasting and go for a whole 48 hours without a meal. For beginners, you can start by having your food at 8 pm, for example, and having nothing again until 8 am the next day. It will be easier since sleep is incorporated into your eating window.

Avoid stress

Intermittent might be hard to do if you are stressed. This is because stress can trigger an overindulgence of food to some people. It is also easier to feed on junk when stressed to feel better. That's why when on intermittent fasting, you are advised to avoid if not control your stress levels.

Be disciplined

Remember that fasting means the abstinence of food until a particular time. When fasting, be true to yourself and avoid eating before the stipulated time. It will ensure that you lose maximum weight and benefit health-wise from intermittent fasting.

Keep off flavored drinks

Most flavored drink says that they are low in sugar, but in the real sense, they are not. Flavored drinks contain artificial sweeteners, which will affect your health negatively. They will also increase your appetite, causing you to overeat, and this will make you gain weight instead of losing.

Find something to do when fasting

It is said that an idle mind is the devil's workshop. When you are on intermittent fasting and not busy, you will be thinking about food, and this will make you break your fast before the stipulated time. You can keep yourself busy by running errands, listening to music, or even taking a walk in the park.

Exercising

Exercise can be done when fasting, but it is not a must. Mild exercises can be done even at home. By exercising, you will build your muscle strength, and your body fat will burn faster.

Chapter 14: Most Common Mistakes and How to Avoid Them

When you are looking to make any significant adjustments in your life, it can take time to discover exactly how to do it in the best ways possible. Many people will make mistakes and have some setbacks as they seek to improve their health through intermittent fasting. Some of these mistakes are minor and can easily be overcome, whereas others may be dangerous and could cause serious repercussions if they are not caught in time.

In this chapter, we are going to explore common mistakes that people tend to make when they are on the intermittent fasting diet. We will also explore why these mistakes are made, and how they can be avoided. It is important that you read through this chapter before you actually commit to the diet itself. That way, you can ensure that you are avoiding any potential mistakes beforehand. This will help you in avoiding unwanted problems and achieving your results with greater success and fewer setbacks.

You should also keep this chapter handy as you embark on your intermittent fasting diet. That way, if you do begin to notice that things are not going as you had hoped, you can easily reflect back on this chapter and get the information that you need to adjust your diet and improve your results.

Switching Too Fast

A significant number of people fail to comply with their new diets because they attempt to go too hard too fast. Trying to jump too quickly can result in you feeling too extreme of a departure from your normal. As a result, both psychologically and physically you are put under a significant amount of stress from your new diet. This can lead to you feeling like the diet is not actually effective and like you are suffering more than you are actually benefitting from it.

If you are someone who eats regularly and who snacks frequently, switching to the intermittent fasting diet will take time and patience. I cannot stress the importance of your transition period enough.

It is not uncommon to want to jump off the deep end when you are making a lifestyle change. Often, we want to experience great results right away and we are excited about the switch. However, after a few days, it can feel stressful. Because you didn't give your mind and body enough time to adapt to the changes, you ditch your new diet in favor of things that are more comfortable.

Fasting is something that should always be acclimated to over a period of time. There is no set period, it needs to be done based on what feels right for you and your body. If you are not properly listening to your body and its needs you are going to end up suffering in major ways. Especially with diets like intermittent fasting, letting yourself adapt to the changes and listening to your body's needs can ensure that you are not neglecting your body in favor of strictly following someone else's guide on what to do.

Choosing the Wrong Plan for Your Lifestyle

It is not uncommon to forget the importance of picking a fasting cycle that actually fits with your lifestyle and then fitting it in. Trying to fast to a cycle that does not fit with your lifestyle will ultimately result in you feeling inconvenienced by your diet and struggling to maintain it.

Often, the way we naturally eat is in accordance with what we feel fits into our lifestyle in the best way possible. So, if you look at your present diet and notice that there are a lot of convenience meals and they happen all throughout the day, you can conclude two things:

138

you are busy, and you eat when you can. Picking a diet that allows you to eat when you can is important in helping you stick to it. It is also important that you begin searching for healthier convenience options so that you can get the most out of your diet.

Anytime you make a lifestyle change, such as with your diet, you need to consider what your lifestyle actually is. In an ideal world, you may be able to adapt everything to suit your dreamy needs completely. However, in the real world, there are likely many aspects of your lifestyle that are not practical to adjust. Picking a diet that suits your lifestyle rather than picking a lifestyle that suits your diet makes far more sense.

Taking the time to actually document what your present eating habits are like before you embark on your intermittent fasting diet is a great way to begin. Focus on what you are already eating and how often and consider diets that will serve your lifestyle. You should also consider your activity levels and how much food you truly need at certain times of the day. For example, if you have a spin class every morning, fasting until noon might not be a good idea as you could end up hungry and exhausted after your class. Choosing the dieting pattern that fits your lifestyle will help you actually maintain your diet so you can continue receiving great results from it.

Eating Too Much or Not Enough

Focusing on what you are eating and how much you are eating is important. This is one of the biggest reasons why a gradual and intentional transition can be helpful. If you are used to eating throughout the entire day, attempting to eat the same amount in a shorter window can be challenging. You may find yourself feeling stuffed and far too full to actually sustain that amount of eating on a day-to-day basis. As a result, you may find yourself not eating enough.

If you are new to intermittent fasting and you take the leap too quickly, it is not unusual to find yourself scarfing down as much food as you possibly can the moment your eating window opens back up. As a result, you find yourself feeling sick, too full, and uncomfortable. Your body also struggles to process and digest that much food after having been fasting for any given period of time. This can be even harder on your body if you have been using a more intense fast and then you stuff yourself. If you find yourself doing this, it may be a sign that you have transitioned too quickly and that you need to slow down and back off.

You might also find yourself not eating enough. Attempting to eat the same amount that you typically eat in 12-16 hours in just 8-12 hours can be challenging. It may not sound so drastic on paper, but if you are not hungry you may simply not feel like eating. As a result, you may feel compelled to skip meals. This can lead to you not getting enough calories and nutrition on a daily basis. In the end, you find yourself not eating enough and feeling unsatisfied during your fasting windows.

The best way to combat this is to begin practicing making calorie-dense foods before you actually start intermittent fasting. Learning what recipes you can make and how much each meal needs to have in order to help you reach your goals is a great way to get yourself ready and show yourself what it truly takes to succeed. Then, begin gradually shortening your eating window and giving yourself the time to work up to eating enough during those eating windows without overeating. In the end, you will find yourself feeling amazing and not feeling unsatisfied or overeating as you maintain your diet.

Your Food Choices are Not Healthy Enough

Even if you are eating according to the keto diet or any other dietary style while you are intermittently fasting, it is not uncommon to find yourself eating the wrong food choices. Simply knowing what to eat and what to avoid is not enough. You need to spend some time getting to understand what specific vitamins, and minerals you need to thrive. That way, you can eat a diet that is rich in these specific nutrients. Then, you can trust that your body has everything that it needs to thrive on your diet.

Even though intermittent fasting does not technically outline what you should and should not eat, it is not a one-size-fits-all diet that can help you lose weight while eating anything you want. In other words, excessive amounts of junk foods will still have a negative impact on you, even if you're eating during the right windows.

It is important that you choose a diet that is going to help you maintain everything you need to function optimally. Ideally, you should combine intermittent fasting with another diet such as the keto diet, the Mediterranean diet, or any other diet that supports you in eating healthfully. Following the guidelines of these healthier diets ensures that you are incorporating the proper nutrients into your diet so that you can stay healthy.

Eating the right nutrients is essential as it will support your body in healthy hormonal balance and bodily functions. This is how you can keep your organs functioning effectively so that everything works the way it should. As a result, you end up feeling healthier and experiencing greater benefits from your diet. It is imperative that you focus on this if you want to have success with your intermittent fasting diet.

You are Not Drinking Enough Fluids

Many people do not realize how much hydration their foods actually give them on a day-to-day basis. Food like fruit and vegetables are filled with hydration that supports your body in healthily functions. If you are not eating as many, then you can guarantee that you are not getting as much hydration as you actually need to be. This means that you need to focus on increasing your hydration levels.

When you are dehydrated you can experience many unwanted symptoms that can make intermittent fasting a challenge. Increased headaches, muscle cramping, and increased hunger are all side effects of dehydration. A great way to combat dehydration is to make sure that you keep water nearby and sip it often. At least once every fifteen minutes to half an hour you should have a good drink of water. This will ensure that you are getting plenty of freshwater into your system.

Other ways that you can maintain your hydration levels include drinking low-calorie sports drinks, bone broth, tea, and coffee. Essentially, drinking low-calorie drinks throughout the course of the entire day can be extremely helpful in supporting your health. Make sure that you do not exceed your fasting calorie maximum, however, or you will stop gaining the benefits of fasting. As well, water should always be your first choice above any other drinks to maintain your hydration. However, including some of the others from time to time can support you and keep things interesting so that you can stay hydrated but not bored.

If you begin to experience any symptoms of dehydration, make sure that you immediately begin increasing the amount of water that you are drinking. Dehydration can lead to far more serious side effects beyond headaches and muscle cramps if you are not careful. If you find that you are prone to not drinking enough water on a daily basis, consider setting a reminder on your phone that keeps you drinking plenty throughout the day.

The best way to tell that you are staying hydrated enough is to pay attention to how frequently you are peeing. If you are staying in a healthy range of hydration, you should be peeing at least once every single hour. If you aren't, this means that you need to be drinking more water, even if you aren't experiencing any side effects of dehydration. Typically, if you have already begun experiencing side effects then you have waited too long. You want to maintain healthy hydration without waiting for symptoms like headaches and muscle aches to inform you that it is time to start drinking more. This ensures that your body stays happy and healthy and that you are not causing unnecessary suffering or stress to your body throughout the day.

You Are Giving Up Too Quickly

A lot of people assume that eating the intermittent fasting diet means that they will see the benefits of their eating habits immediately. This is not the case. While intermittent fasting does typically offer great results fairly quickly, it does take some time for these results to begin appearing. The exact amount of time depends on many factors. How long it has taken you to transition, what and how you are eating during eating windows, and how much activity you are getting throughout the day all contribute to your results.

You might feel compelled to quickly give up if you do not begin noticing your desired results right away, but trust that this is not going to help you. Some people require several weeks before they really begin seeing the benefits of their dieting. This does not mean that it is not working, it simply means that it has taken them some time to find the right balance so that they can gain their desired results and stay healthy.

If you are feeling like throwing in the towel, first take a few minutes to consider what you are doing and how it may be negatively impacting your results. A great way to do this is to try using your food diary once again. For a few days, track how you are eating in accordance with the intermittent fasting diet and what it is doing for you. Get a clear idea of how much you are eating, what you are eating, and when you are eating it. Also, track the amount of physical activity that you are doing on a daily basis.

Through tracking your food intake and exercise levels, you might find that you are not experiencing the results you desire because you are eating too much or not enough in comparison to the amount of energy you are spending each day. Then, you can easily work towards adjusting your diet to find a balance that supports you in getting everything you need and also seeing the results that you desire.

In most cases, intermittent fasting diets are not working because they are not being used right for the individual person. Although the general requirements are somewhat the same, each of us has unique needs based on our lifestyles and our unique makeup. If you are willing to invest time in finding the right balance for yourself then you can guarantee that you can overcome this and experience great results from your fasting.

You Are Getting Too Intense or Pushing It

If you are really focused on achieving your desired results, you might feel compelled to push your diet further than what is reasonable for you. For example, attempting to take on too intense of a fasting cycle or trying to do more than your body can reasonably handle. It is not uncommon for people to try and push themselves beyond reasonable measures to achieve their desired results. Unfortunately, this rarely results in them achieving what they actually set out to achieve. It can also have severe consequences.

At the end of the day, listening to your body and paying attention to exactly what it needs is important. You need to be taking care of yourself through proper nutrition and proper exercise levels. You also need to balance these two in a way that serves your body, rather than in a way that leads to you feeling sick and unwell. If you push your body too far, the negative consequences can be severe and long-lasting. In some cases, they may even be life-threatening.

In some cases, pushing your body to a certain extent is necessary. For example, if you are seeking to build more muscle then you want to push yourself to work out enough that your workouts are actually effective. However, if you are pushing yourself to the point that you are beginning to experience negative side effects from your diet, you need to drawback. While certain amounts of side effects are fairly normal early on, experiencing intense side effects, having side effects that don't go away, or having them return is not good. You want to work towards maintaining and minimizing your side effects, not constantly living alongside them. After all, what is the point of adjusting your diet and lifestyle to serve your health if you are not actually feeling healthy while you do it?

144

Make sure that you check in with yourself on a daily basis to see to it that your physical needs are being met. That way, if anything begins to feel excessive or any symptoms begin to increase, you can focus on minimizing or eliminating them right away. Paying close attention to your needs and looking at your goals long-term rather than trying to reach them immediately is the best way to ensure that you reach your health goals without actually compromising your health while attempting to do so. In the end, you will feel much better about doing it this way.

Chapter 15: The Right Mindset

We all know in the 21st century that wellbeing starts with healthy eating habits. Then why is it so difficult to stick to a balanced diet? The grocery store's aisles, posters on the doctor's offices, and even some TV advertisements use vivid colors and bold lettering to advertise healthy living. Women over 50 years are especially advised to watch what they eat as it is easier for them to gain weight than lose it.

The issue is not because people don't want to change their eating habits; it's that they don't even know how to do it. They get on board a new weight-loss plan, which they soon discard as such diets are often unsustainable when compared with regular lifestyles.

That's not the best way to go for a balanced lifestyle. Instead, you want to make a meaningful, permanent improvement, but you have to make sure you are doing it right. The guide below will help and show you how to stick to healthy eating habits. By setting realistic expectations and being persistent, you will find that good eating patterns are now well within your grasp even though they were impossible in the past. Each diet and weight-loss plan has its benefits and drawbacks, so you have to prepare your mind for it if you want to succeed.

The hardest factor in weight loss is changing your attitude about how to lose weight.

Many people attempt to lose weight with the worst imaginable mental state. They bolt into diets and workout programs out of personal-deprecation, all the while squeezing their "trouble" spots, branding themselves "fat" and feeling entirely less than that. They get distracted with results, rely on fast solutions, and lose sight of what good health is all about.

This kind of thought can be harmful. Instead of concentrating on the benefits that can come from weight loss—such as improved wellbeing, healthier life, greater satisfaction of daily lives, and the avoidance of diabetes and cardiac disease—these people focus on their pessimistic feelings. Eventually, poor thinking leads to disappointment.

Changing your mentality about weight loss goes beyond feeling-good; it's about the outcome. A study at the University of Syracuse indicates that the more unhappy women are with their bodies, the more likely they are to skip exercise. And just focusing on the fact that you're overweight is forecasting a potential weight gain—according to studies reported in the International Journal of Obesity in 2015.

Although psychologists emphasize that your actions are determined by how you view yourself and your core personality (seeing yourself as being overweight or undesirable makes you behave accordingly), genetics may also play a role. A study published in Psychosomatic Medicine journal also suggested that cortisol, the stress hormone, is secreted by the adrenal glands every time you get yourself down or think about your weight, which further causes weight gain.

It All Starts With Your Mindset

The problem with a lot of trendy diets is that they don't want you to think differently. They tell you to make a drastic adjustment to your eating habits. This is not healthy. If you are actively trying to change your eating habits, then first you have to fix your way of thinking about food.

Many people who are struggling to eat healthily have what researchers term a "closed mentality." These people believe that nothing can ever change, and they take this belief with them in beginning a new weight loss plan. They think that their health issues are simply the effects of poor biology, or that the embarrassment of solving the problem would reverse any improvements.

For certain people with a fixed mentality, long before it begins, a change of diet is futile. In reality, many would prefer to stay obese because it feels safer and less stressful than attempting to make a lifestyle change.

Unfortunately, anyone who wants to move to a healthier lifestyle without changing their attitude first will soon get discouraged. That's because the journey to a healthy lifestyle doesn't happen overnight. There are no magic foods, no matter what the magazine said or what some star did to shed baby weight or to dress for a new role. If you are someone with a fixed mindset starting a weight loss diet, you'll undoubtedly come to think the plan failed when you don't see any significant difference—reinforcing your original fears. The diet's failure will only make it harder for you to begin a new journey to eating healthy. There is another mindset that Psychologists refer to as a "growth mindset." While the fixed mindset believes little else can be changed, the growth mindset thinks things are continually evolving.

People with a growth mindset don't design their thoughts to be negative. Instead, they understand that small mistakes are just part of improvement. They realize that risks are only a minor problem in achieving something big. Therefore, people with a growth mindset recognize that progress needs incremental steps in the right direction, rather than resigning themselves to the inevitable.

What kind of attitude do you have? If you have a fixed mindset, how do you make the necessary change?

One of the easiest ways to begin making a change is by collecting information about the process. I highly recommend that you maintain a journal. This is so when you see subtle improvements leading up to a significant transition, they don't get lost. Start by writing down your expectations and record whether or not you have successfully met them.

A growth mindset is not a crazy dreamer mindset when it comes to goals. When setting your targets, always make sure that they are fair. Keep note of how many balanced meals you consume, relative to how many might not be. Act to increase the number of nutritious meals you consume each week.

You've got to understand more than anything that your mindset may be what held you off. The good news is that you're well on your way to make a meaningful difference when you know that mindset is part of the problem!

Below are some steps you can take to change your mindset.

Adjust your Priorities

The reason might be to lose weight, but that should not be the target. Instead, the objectives should be small, manageable stuff that you have full power to control. Have you consumed five fruit and veggie servings today? That's one goal achieved. What about 8 hours of sleep; have you got them in? If so, you can cross them off your list.

Gravitate to Positivity

It is vital to Surround yourself with the Good. Doing so offers you a relaxing, socially healthy environment to invest in yourself. Don't be afraid to ask for help or support.

Rethink Punishments and Rewards

Remember that making healthier decisions is a way to practice self-care. Food is not a reward, and a workout is not a penalty. They are all necessary to take care of your body and to make you do the best you can. You deserve both.

Taking a few minutes at the start of your exercise or at the beginning of your day to calm down, and simply concentrate on breathing will help you set your goals, communicate with your body, and even reduce the stress response of your body.

Find a quiet space wherever you are (even at work), and try this exercise to help you feel more relaxed and ready to tackle the rest of your day. Lie with your legs outstretched on your back and put one hand on your stomach and one on your shoulder. Breathe in for four seconds through your nose, stay for two, and exhale for six seconds through your lips. Repeat this process for 5-10 minutes, focusing on the sensation of your stomach rising and falling with each breath.

24 Hour Goals

Having patience is essential when you are losing weight. Plus, if you concentrate on reaching genuinely reachable targets, such as taking 10.000 steps each day, you don't need to be caught up in your list of goals. New accomplishments come in every 24 hours; concentrate on those.

Like Bob Proctor says: "If you want to improve the quality of your life, start allocating a portion of each day to changing your paradigm."

Identify 'Troublesome Thoughts'

Identify the feelings that bring you problems, and seek to prevent and change them. Let them stop intentionally by saying 'no' out loud. It may sound silly, but that simple action breaks your chain of thought and helps you to introduce a new, safer one. The easiest way to do so is to count as many times as you like from one to 100 until your negative thoughts go away.

Don't step on the scale

Even though stepping on the scale to check on your progress is not bad, many people often associate it with negative thoughts. If you know the number on the scale will lead to negative and self-destructive thoughts, then you should avoid it. At least until you are in a place where the number on the scale doesn't affect your mental health.

Forget about the Entire 'Foods' attitude

We've learned somewhere along the way to feel either proud or bad for any food choice we make. But in the end, it's just food, so you shouldn't feel bad for enjoying an occasional cookie. Permit yourself to have a piece of chocolate cake or a glass of wine sometimes.

Treating yourself to some comfort food is right for your mind and body. It is doing it every day that sabotages weight loss. During a more or less strict diet, having a day in a week to get away from is the key to success, the guarantee for motivation, and does not undermine the goal of losing weight.

Focus on the Attainable

If you've never been to a gym before, your goal on day one shouldn't be to do 30 minutes on the elliptical. Going for a 30-minute walk might be a better goal. If you want to cook more but have little familiarity with healthier cooking, don't bank on creating new nutritious recipes every night after work. Instead, consider using a subscription service such as Blue Apron or HelloFresh, where pre-portioned recipes and ingredients are delivered to your doorstep, helping you get to know different components, make new meals, and develop your cooking skills.

Envision a better life

What will life be like if you put good habits in place? Will you be more comfortable in your clothes? Will it give you more energy? Will you sleep better? Will you laugh more? Will you be happier? Will you be a better wife or mum? Attempt to get as thorough and realistic as possible. How will your life change if you changed your lifestyle?

Take a moment and sit down with a pen and ask yourself, what do I want? What do I really want? Write it down and make a written description of it in the present tense. Build a vision of what you would like to accomplish.

Take time to visualize a better life in the beginning and throughout your weight loss plan. Changing your habits is hard, so why bother if it doesn't bring you something new and better. Imagine a better life that will start giving you something to look forward to as well as work towards. See what you want, get a picture of it in your mind. Vision is going to direct your life.

Believe in your vision

This is important. There's no point in having a vision unless you think it will come true. With almost everything, you have to believe that you can make this happen. So you can change your lifestyle, lose weight, and hope for a better future. To be successful, you have to believe you can do it without anybody else's evaluation. You have to believe in what you see. Keep your vision up front, and think it's waiting for you. You have to persist and persevere in working on what you want to achieve. That'll keep you focused and move on.

Imagining a happier future makes you hopeful – although things go wrong sometimes, you will just have to hope it's for the greater good. Learning not to focus on the bad will help you stay focused on living a healthier lifestyle.

Sacrifice is giving up something of a lower nature, to receive something of a higher nature. Sacrifice is based on faith, and if you have faith, you will take action.

Believe you are in control

You must realize you control your life. You have to take responsibility for your actions to excel in losing weight and other goals – you have to trust that you are in charge. If you put your future in other people's hands, you will never be able to move on. Of course, there are always circumstances out of our control, but your type of reaction is up to you.

While taking control of your life is empowering, it's also frightening because if you don't achieve your goal, you have no one to blame but yourself. "No one has control over your life – but you."

Get to learn how to cope

Many of your problems with weight loss are from your physiological reactions to stress. Most times, you crave spaghetti or candy when you have a bad day. Or you order a pizza because there was nothing to cook for dinner. Or give up on losing weight when work gets busy, or when you get to some other stressful season of life.

When you want to lose weight, life doesn't just continue effortlessly without stress. Sadly, life will never be secure, and there will always be a pain. Consequently, if you fall off track each time, life does not go your way, then it is time you learn new coping strategies. The goal is to maintain a healthy lifestyle and lose weight, no matter the obstacles life throws our way.

If the way you cope with stress keeps you from putting new behaviors in place or maintaining them, you might want to talk to a therapist or counselor. A therapist or psychologist will help you develop healthier coping skills and work through stress. This will help you free up space in your brain to focus on that better life. Having excellent optimistic coping skills is necessary for growth and surviving – not just for weight loss. Life is unpredictable and will not always go according to plan. Either you can get better or get bitter.

"The secret of success is learning how to use pain and pleasure instead of having pain and pleasure use you. If you do that, you're in control of your life. If you don't, life controls you." Tony Robbins

Eliminate the clutter and the chaos

What do clutter and chaos have to do with weight loss? It's tough to picture a happier future when you are surrounded by confusion and noise. Clutter and confusion build hot zones, and when attempting to escape hot zones, it's challenging to develop new patterns and behaviors. Hot zones are moments when you feel stressed, overwhelmed, and th

e decisions you make are more about surviving the moment than on long-term goals.

Concentrate on solutions and not explanations

A proactive approach that has been effective in the weight loss process is relying on options instead of excuses. You may be using excuses because you're scared of failing. So you say something like, "I can't get to the gym at that time" or "I 'm sick" or "That exercise never worked for me" instead of falling into an exercise routine. It offers you the freedom to either give up or not try at all. Failure, however, is part of the process. Failure is Good. And instead of making yourself give up, grant yourself the approval to lose. To succeed, you have to be okay with failure, not just at losing weight but in life in general.

Chapter 16: Useful Supplements – Spirulina Algae

Spirulina (pronounced speer-uh-lee-nuh) is an edible type of cyanobacteria, a single-celled, blue-green microalgae that is found naturally in both salt and freshwaters. This spiral-shaped microalga is cultivated and harvested throughout the world as both a supplement and whole food. Because it has a soft cell wall made of protein and complex sugars, it can be digested efficiently. It is widely considered a green superfood with positive health benefits because of its richness in:

- Protein (dried spirulina contains between 50% to 70% protein)

- Minerals (especially Iron and Manganese)

- Vitamins (especially Vitamins B1, and B2)

- Carotenoids

- Antioxidants

Spirulina is used internationally in nutrition drinks, pasta, crackers, noodles, nutrition bars, broths, cakes, pet foods, and cereal. It is also used as a component in food coloring, cosmetics, skin creams, shampoos, personal care products, and more. Spirulina can be purchased at most specialty nutrition stores, some supermarket chains, as well as online. It is typically sold in powder or tablet form.

As a food, eating spirulina is nothing new. Historians indicate that spirulina was part of the diet of the Kanem Empire of Chad in the ninth century (AD/CE). In 1519, Hernando Cortez and his Spanish Conquistadors observed that spirulina was eaten by Aztecs around Lake Texcoco, which is modern-day Mexico City. Today, more than one thousand metric tons of spirulina are harvested worldwide in natural lakes, commercial farms, village farms, and family microfarms.

Spirulina farming is much more environmentally friendly compared to conventional food production. Most conventional foods are generated using chemicals including pesticides, antibiotics, preservatives, additives, and fungicides. Not only have these chemicals been shown to have negative impacts on health, but they also cause damage to our water supply and the overall natural environment. Harvesting spirulina offers more nutrition per acre, and doesn't incur environmental costs associated with toxic cleanup, water treatment, or subsidies, that other food industries require.

The growing popularity of spirulina as a green superfood has taken off over the past forty years. Scientific research conducted in recent decades support the many health benefits of spirulina, adding to its growing use as a food or supplement. Research is ongoing, and in some cases, has not been tested on human subjects. Additionally, the U.S. FDA has not approved spirulina as a medicine or treatment for diseases (although it is an approved supplement and food). However, the health benefits that research has uncovered so far have been very positive, showing some transformative results.

Cancer Fighter

Spirulina is high in beta-carotene, a type of phytochemical, that is believed to help protect the body against free radicals that can come from various forms of pollution including cigarette smoke and herbicides. The effects of spirulina on cancer have been demonstrated in animals and humans with positive effects indicating a reduction in cancer cells, and even in some cases, the reversal of oral cancer.

Diabetes and Blood Sugar Improvement

A study from the University of Baroda in India revealed that spirulina may help people with diabetes. Over the course of a two-month study, patients with type 2 diabetes who were given two grams of spirulina every day improved blood sugar and lipid levels.

Immune System Boost

Tests on animals and senior citizens have exhibited a boost of the immune system, which is crucial to preventing viral infections. In these studies, spirulina was shown to increase the production of antibodies, which are needed to fight viral and bacterial infections, as well as some chronic illnesses.

Anti-Virus

Not only has the algae been observed to boos antibodies, but it has also shown an ability to hinder the replication of viruses. The National Cancer Institute (NCI) publicized that spirulina was "remarkably active" against the AIDS virus (HIV-1) after conducting a study in 1989. Test tube experiments have also shown spirulina to inhibit the replication of other viruses including influenza A, mumps, and measles.

Antihistamine

In several scientific studies, spirulina appeared to help allergy symptoms such as watery eyes, skin reactions, and runny nose. In a recent study, a group of people suffering from rhinitis, an inflammation of the nasal mucous membrane, saw significant improvements in their allergy symptoms when given a daily 1000mg or 2000mg doses of spirulina over the course of twelve weeks.

Blood Pressure Reduction

Participants in an experiment at the National Autonomous University of Mexico were able to drop their blood pressure after taking spirulina for six weeks, without any other changes in their diet. Spirulina increases the body's production of nitric oxide, which is a gas that can widen blood vessels. Widened blood vessels improve the body's flow of blood, and ultimately can reduce blood pressure.

Lower Cholesterol

Recent research conducted in Greek universities has shown some promising effects on adults with high cholesterol. Over the course of three months, fifty-two adults were given one gram of spirulina each day. At the end of the three-month study period, the group's average triglycerides decreased over 16% and low-density lipoprotein (LDL) cholesterol (also known as the "bad" cholesterol) by 10%.

Radiation Treatment

After the Russian Chernobyl nuclear disaster in 1986, the Russian government turned to spirulina to treat children who had been exposed to radiation. Radiation destroys bone marrow, thus complicating the body's ability to create normal white or red blood cells. Within six weeks, children who were fed five grams of spirulina every day were able to make remarkable recoveries. The blue pigment of spirulina is comprised of phycocyanin, which enables the body to cleanse some radioactive metals.

Kidney and Liver Detoxification

Not only has spirulina's phycocyanin been shown to cleanse radioactive metals, but it may also have the ability to cleanse heavy metal poisoning. Studies in Japan and elsewhere suggest that spirulina is able to safely assist in the removal of heavy metals such as arsenic, lead, mercury, and other similar metals that can be found in medicine, dental fillings, fish, deodorants, cigarettes, and drinking water.

Reducing Malnutrition

According to the United Nations Food and Agricultural Organization, over 800 million people worldwide suffer from chronic undernourishment. Malnutrition is an epidemic as millions of people around the world lack enough proteins and micronutrients such as vitamins and minerals. With spirulina containing a significant amount of protein, B-vitamins, and iron, one tablespoon a day could eliminate micronutrient deficiencies that cause diseases such as anemia. Unlike other protein foods such as beef or nuts, spirulina is a very digestible source of protein. The digestive tract of malnourished individuals exhibits malabsorption, making the easily digestible spirulina, an even more attractive source of nourishment.

Conclusion

As you can see, there are numerous benefits that come with employing an intermittent fasting diet. After reading this book, you now have this information and much, much more! You are fully equipped to begin changing your life with programs designed specifically for you, and I hope that you feel empowered to do so!

The main takeaway from this book is that there are many options for women over the age of 50 to take control of their weight loss strategies without having to turn to methods designed for men or people in their twenties. Further, taking control of your health and playing an active role in your disease risk reduction is not as difficult as it sounds. I hope that after reading this book, you have a new understanding of what you can do and how your body will react, given your age and sex.

As you take all of this information forth with you, it may seem overwhelming to begin applying this to your own life. Remember, life is a process, and you do not need to expect perfection from yourself. By reading this book, you are already on your way to changing your life. If you fall off of the diet and you need inspiration, come back to the first chapters of this book and remind yourself why you wanted to begin it in the first place.

Many thanks for completing this book. I hope it was practical enough and able to provide you with the vital tools you need to attain your fitness goals.

CPSIA information can be obtained
at www.ICGtesting.com
Printed in the USA
LVHW061500030621
689276LV00003B/308

9 781914 373909